MICROBIOLOGY AND IMMUNOLOGY

for the
Boards and Wards

D1431235

Don't miss other books in Blackwell's *Boards and Wards* series!

Behavioral Science for the Boards and Wards

Boards and Wards, 2e

Dermatology for the Boards and Wards

Ophthalmology and Otolaryngology for the Boards and Wards

Pathophysiology for the Boards and Wards, 4e

Pharmacology for the Boards and Wards

MICROBIOLOGY AND IMMUNOLOGY

for the

Boards and Wards

Carlos Ayala, MD
Otolaryngology Head & Neck Surgery
MacDill AFB, FL

Brad Spellberg, MD
Assistant Professor of Medicine
Geffen School of Medicine at UCLA
Division of Infectious Diseases
Harbor-UCLA Medical Center
Torrance, CA

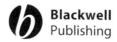

Blackwell
Publishing

Blackwell Publishing, Inc., 350 Main Street, Malden, Massachusetts 02148-5018, USA
Blackwell Publishing Ltd, 9600 Garsington Road, Oxford OX4 2DQ, UK
Blackwell Publishing Asia Pty Ltd, 550 Swanston Street, Carlton, Victoria 3053, Aus

**QW
18.2
A973m
2005**

05 06 07 08 5 4 3 2 1

ISBN-13: 978-1-4051-0468-5
ISBN-10: 1-4051-0468-6

Library of Congress Cataloging-in-Publication Data
Ayala, Carlos, MD.
    Microbiology and immunology for the boards and wards / authors, Carlos Ayala, Brad Spellberg.
        p. ; cm.–(Blackwell's boards and wards series)
    Includes index.
    ISBN-10: 1-4051-0468-6 (pbk.)
    ISBN-13: 978-1-4051-0468-5 (pbk.)
    1. Microbiology–Outlines, syllabi, etc. 2. Microbiology–Examinations, questions, etc.
    3. Immunology–Outlines, syllabi, etc. 4. Immunology–Examinations, questions, etc.
    [DNLM: 1. Microbiology–Examination Questions. 2. Immune System Diseases–Examination
    Questions. 3. Immunity–Examination Questions. QW 18.2 A973m 2005] I. Spellberg, Brad. II.
    Title. III. Series: Boards and wards series.
QR62.A97 2005
616.9'041—dc22   2004029351

A catalogue record for this title is available from the British Library

Acquisitions: Beverly Copland
Development: William Deluise
Production: Jennifer Kowalewski
Typesetter: International Typesetting and Composition in India
Printed and bound by Edwards Brother in Ann Arbor, MI

For further information on Blackwell Publishing, visit our website:
www.blackwellmedstudent.com

Notice: The indications and dosages of all drugs in this book have been recommended in the medical literature and conform to the practices of the general
community. The medications described do not necessarily have specific approval by
the Food and Drug Administration for use in the diseases and dosages for which
they are recommended. The package insert for each drug should be consulted for
use and dosage as approved by the FDA. Because standards for usage change, it is
advisable to keep abreast of revised recommendations, particularly those concern-
ing new drugs.

The publisher's policy is to use permanent paper from mills that operate a sustain-
able forestry policy, and which has been manufactured from pulp processed using
acid-free and elementary chlorine-free practices. Furthermore, the publisher ensures
that the text paper and cover board used have met acceptable environmental
accreditation standards.

CONTENTS

TABLES

FIGURES

ABBREVIATIONS

↑↓	increases or high/decreases or low
→	causes, leads to, analysis shows
CXR	chest x-ray
CNS	central nervous system
Dx	diagnosis
dz	disease
1°/2°	primary/secondary
GNC	gram negative cocci
GNR	gram negative rods
GPC	gram positive cocci
GPR	gram positive rods
hr(s)	hour(s)
Ig	immunoglobin
IL	interleukin
infxn	infection
lmtd	limited
pt(s)	patient(s)
Tx	treatment
μg	microgram
μL	microliter
μm	micrometer
WBC	white blood cells
yr(s)	year(s)

PREFACE

A number of medical students have told us how useful they have found our *Boards and Wards* review book for clerkship and the USMLE Steps 2 & 3, as well as our *Pathophysiology for the Boards and Wards*, for their USMLE Step 1 review. With that in mind, we set out to create a combined microbiology and immunology review book that addresses the most essential information that medical students encounter in microbiology and immunology courses, and on the USMLE Step 1.

In this book, we maintain our outline format to spare readers needless information and to save time for busy medical students and interns who need a quick, ready reference for review. Our goal was to make this book the perfect complement for busy students and housestaff, and we hope that we've succeeded.

The microbiology section contains descriptions of microorganisms, broken into eight categories: appearance, lab assays, virulence factors, epidemiology, clinical diseases, treatment, resistance, and prophylaxis. We do not intend a complete microbiological description of each pathogen. Instead, we provide information in each category only as it relates to testable USMLE material. Thus, you will frequently see "none" or "none significant" listed under the virulence factor section. This doesn't literally mean that there are no virulence factors associated with the organism. Instead, it means there are no virulence factors you will be asked about on the Boards exam. At the end of each section of organisms (e.g., gram positive cocci), we include summary tables listing the key characteristics of each organism for ease of rapid review.

The description of antibiotics is similarly broken into five sections, including mechanism, resistance, toxicities, cidal/static, and spectrum of coverage. Again, we focus only on information that is important for the USMLE exams.

In the immunology section, we view the immune system from the perspective of a host organism assigned the task of defending itself from a hostile, microbe-infested environment. This section focuses on what really happens inside the body during an infection, from the assigned duties of each of the types of immune cells, to the arsenals they have at their disposal, to the cooperative defensive structures of immune organs and tissues.

At the end of each section, we have included 25 questions with complete answer explanations. These are designed to allow you to review content as you complete each of the sections. At the end of the book appears a self-assessment test of 50 questions and answers, further allowing you to evaluate your understanding of the content of this book.

We are confident that you will find this book useful for your preparation for the boards and wards. Good luck to all of you!

ACKNOWLEDGMENTS

The authors would like to offer their most sincere thanks to Dr. Samuel French, Professor of Pathology at the Geffen School of Medicine at UCLA and the Harbor-UCLA Department of Pathology. Dr. French provided all of the microbiology images for this book. He is a paragon of academic excellence, a true gentleman and scholar, who has throughout his career selflessly taught innumerable residents and students.

We would like to thank the great staff at Blackwell Publishing, Beverly Copland and Laura DeYoung in particular, for their many years of dedication to us and the Boards & Wards series.

REVIEWERS

Bob Armin
Class of 2006
David Geffen School of Medicine, UCLA
Los Angeles, California

Filip Bednar
Class of 2006
Temple University School of Medicine
Philadelphia, Pennsylvania

Amberly Burger
Class of 2006
Ohio State University College of Medicine and Public Health
Columbus, Ohio

Patricia Frew
Class of 2007
Oregon Health & Science University, School of Medicine
Portland, Oregon

John Froelich
Class of 2006
Southern Illinois University School of Medicine
Springfield, Illinois

Serge Hougeir
Class of 2006
University of Arizona College of Medicine
Phoenix, Arizona

Jared Jagdeo
Class of 2006
Brown Medical School
Providence, Rhode Island

Ray Jalian
Class of 2006
David Geffen School of Medicine, UCLA
Los Angeles, California

Michelle Klein
Class of 2005
Marquette University, Physician Assistant Program
Milwaukee, Wisconsin

Adam Kotowski
Class of 2006
School of Medicine and Biomedical Sciences
University at Buffalo, State University of New York
Buffalo, New York

Tanisha Osbourne-Williams
Class of 2006
Howard University College of Medicine
Washington, DC

Fatima Cody Stanford
Class of 2007
Medical College of Georgia
School of Medicine
Augusta, Georgia

Microbiology

I. BASIC CONCEPTS

A. Bacteria

1. **Bacteria are prokaryotes**: single-cell organisms having no internal organelles

2. Almost all bacteria have cell walls, which are thick structures **composed of a cross-linked glycopeptide called peptidoglycan**, providing support for the cell

3. Bacteria also have an outer lipid envelope surrounding the cell wall, **composed of a glycolipid conjugate called lipopolysaccharide (LPS)**

4. Gram stain

    a. The Gram stain is a 2-step process capable of staining different bacteria either purple or red depending upon the type of cell wall and lipid envelope surrounding the cell

    b. In step 1, a purple dye is added to the bacteria which is avidly adherent to the peptidoglycan of the cell wall, and then alcohol is added to wash away non-adherent purple dye

    c. In step 2, a red stain is added to the bacteria

    d. Gram-positive organisms have thick peptidoglycan walls that avidly bind the purple dye, and which do not release the dye when alcohol is added

    e. Gram-negative organisms have thin peptidoglycan walls that are rinsed clean of the purple dye by the alcohol, allowing the cells to be colored by the red counter-stain

    f. **Thus gram-positive organisms stain purple, while gram-negative organisms stain red**

5. Some bacteria have outer polysaccharide capsules surrounding the LPS envelope, which typically serve to protect the bacteria from host immune cells

6. **Atypical bacteria are those that cannot be identified by Gram staining**

7. **Many atypical bacteria are "intracellular pathogens,"** meaning they live inside human cells, which enables them to cause disease

8. Intracellular pathogens have altered cell wall and envelope structures, some have unique lipids called mycolic acids (*Mycobacterium*), and some have no cell walls at all (*Mycoplasma*)

9. **Another kind of atypical bacteria are the spirochetes**, long, spiral-shaped bacteria which move with a corkscrew motion and tend to be extracellular pathogens

10. Flagella are long processes composed of microtubules that extend from the end of a bacterium, which are powered by ATP and are capable of making rapid, whip-like motions to propel the bacterium forward

11. Fimbriae are long glycoprotein extensions from the cell membrane that serve as adhesins to host surfaces, allowing bacterial colonization of a host

12. Infection versus colonization

    a. **Colonization is the peaceful coexistence of bacteria with a mammalian host,** for example *Staphylococcus aureus* living as a commensal organism on our skin

    b. Infection represents an invasive, damaging process initiated by the bacteria, for example cellulitis

    c. It can be very difficult in some clinical situations to determine whether a bacterium is only colonizing a host, and therefore does not need to be treated with antibiotics, or whether it is causing actual disease

    d. **The most reliable marker for infection versus colonization is the host inflammatory response,** that is, bacteria are present in both situations, but host inflammation is only present in infection, not in colonization

B. Fungi

1. **Fungi are eukaryotes,** meaning they have a nucleus and internal organelles separated from the cytoplasm by internal membranes

2. **Fungi all have cell walls,** often composed of complex glycoproteins such as chitin and mannoprotein

3. The chemical composition of fungal cell membranes is distinct from animal cell membranes: **while animal cell membranes contain cholesterol, fungal cell membranes contain ergosterol**

4. Some fungi grow as yeast, which are unicellular spherical forms that reproduce by budding

5. Other fungi grow as molds, which are conglomerates of multicellular, long, filamentous forms called hyphae

6. Still other fungi are called dimorphic because they can grow as yeast or molds depending upon the environment

7. Like a Gram stain for bacteria, **the most useful laboratory stain for detecting fungi is the silver stain**—on a silver stain the background tissue appears light blue-green, while the fungi stain dark black

C. Protozoa

1. **Protozoa are unicellular eukaryotes** of the kingdom Protista

2. **Medically important protozoa are all parasites, meaning they live in humans and cause disease** (as opposed to commensal organisms which live on or in humans but do not cause disease)

3. Protozoa do not have cell walls

4. Many protozoa have complex life cycles involving phase changes in their cellular structure

5. Trophozoites are the forms of protozoa which are motile, whereas cysts are their tough stationary-phase form which allow them to survive in harsh external environments

D. Helminths

1. **Helminths are worms** of the kingdom animalia

2. Helminths are thus **multicellular animals**, and the medically important ones are also parasites

3. Helminths can be divided into flatworms (platyhelminths, platy- = flat) and roundworms (nematodes)

4. Flatworms can be further divided into flukes (also called trematodes) and tapeworms (cestodes)

5. The stool ova and parasite (O&P) test is the classic way to identify worms in an infected patient

E. Viruses

1. Viruses are non-living automatons that hijack living cells and force cellular machinery to replicate the virus

2. Viruses contain a genome composed of RNA or DNA, a variety of structural proteins that form the viral core and viral capsid, and some contain lipid envelopes

3. Viral RNA can either be double-stranded or single-stranded in the viral genome, and single-stranded RNA can either be positive strand or negative strand

    a. Positive strand viral RNA directly codes for viral proteins (equivalent to mRNA)

    b. Negative strand viral RNA must be replicated to the complementary positive strand before transcription is possible

    c. Thus viruses whose genomes consist of negative strand RNA must carry within the viral capsid an RNA polymerase to convert the negative strand to a positive strand if viral replication is to occur

   d. Retroviruses have RNA genomes but convert the RNA into DNA prior to viral replication

   e. Thus, like negative-strand RNA viruses, retroviruses also carry a special viral polymerase, called reverse transcriptase, within their capsid

4. Viral susceptibility to sterilizing agents such as alcohol and halogenated chemicals depends on the presence or absence of the viral envelope

5. Non-enveloped viruses (called naked viruses) are highly resistant to chemical destruction, while enveloped viruses are more susceptible

II. BACTERIA

A. Gram Positive Cocci (GPC)

1. *Staphylococcus*
    a. *S. aureus*
        1) Appearance: **GPC in clusters** ("staphylo-" means "grape-like" in Greek, refers to classic grape-cluster appearance), on Petri dish **colonies have golden hue** (hence *aureus*, which is "gold" in Latin)
        2) Lab assays: **coagulase positive** (secretes coagulase enzyme → clots serum), catalase positive (secretes catalase enzyme → $H_2O_2 \rightarrow H_2O + O_2$), β-hemolytic (see Section 2. *Streptococci*)
        3) Virulence factors:
            a) Protein A is a cell-wall protein that binds to the constant region of IgG antibodies, preventing their variable regions from binding antigen
            b) Enterotoxin (an exotoxin, which is a toxin secreted by bacteria to cause its effect, that is specifically secreted into the gut, or enteric system)
                i)   Pre-formed exotoxin secreted in the intestines (entero = gut), heat resistant
                ii) Causes food-poisoning gastroenteritis, typified by nausea, vomiting, diarrhea, **within 8 hr of food consumption**
                iii) One variant is the Toxic Shock Syndrome Toxin (TSST)
                    a)) A superantigen, binds to a constant region of the T cell receptor, non-specifically activating T lymphocytes resulting in unregulated inflammation
                    b)) Acquired from contaminated tampons in menstruating women or from infected wounds
                    c)) Leads to systemic hypotension, tachycardia
            c) Exfoliation
                i) Also a superantigen, causes "*Staphylococcus* Scalded Skin Syndrome" (SSSS), widespread superficial epidermal exfoliation seen almost exclusively in children
                ii) **Of little clinical consequence**, exfoliation is too superficial to be dangerous, and SSSS resolves quickly with antibiotics
        4) Epidemiology: human skin flora, colonizes the nares, intertriginous areas, and areas of diseased skin such as psoriatic patches, transmission by direct contact and fomites
        5) Clinical Diseases:
            a) Skin infections: include cellulitis, folliculitis, local skin abscess (i.e., furuncle/carbuncle)

b) Bacteremia: **commonly due to intravenous drug abuse (IVDA), post-surgical, via wounds, or nosocomial via intravenous catheters**

c) Endocarditis: causes **acute, severe disease NOT subacute indolent disease**

d) Osteomyelitis

e) Pneumonia: **classically seen during the resolution phase of a prior viral pneumonia,** the patient is getting better and then all of a sudden relapses with severe cough and fevers, **multilobar pneumonia can also be seen in endocarditis due to septic emboli**

6) Treatment:

a) Antibiotic choice depends on whether *S. aureus* is methicillin-susceptible (MSSA) or resistant (MRSA: labs now test for oxacillin susceptibility in lieu of methicillin, as methicillin was taken off the market years ago for high incidence of interstitial nephritis; the name MRSA is a historical throwback, technically it should be called ORSA)

b) For MSSA the drug of choice is a β-lactamase resistant penicillin (e.g., oxacillin/nafcillin), with a second line choice being 1st generation cephalosporin (i.e., cefazolin)—vancomycin is INFERIOR to oxacillin/nafcillin and cefazolin for treatment of MSSA, as vancomycin is only semi-cidal

c) For MRSA, vancomycin has been the workhorse drug for many years, but alternatives are now available, including linezolid (static, oral, hematotoxicities), daptomycin (the most cidal *Staph.* agent of all, IV only), and even trimethoprim-sulfamethoxazole or clindamycin for many strains (see Resistance below)

7) Resistance:

a) β-lactamase: a ubiquitous plasmid-encoded enzyme that inactivates the β-lactam ring common to all penicillins, treatment requires use of a β-lactamase resistant penicillin (e.g., oxacillin/nafcillin), 1st generation cephalosporin, or ampicillin/amoxicillin with addition of a β-lactamase inhibitor (e.g., ampicillin-sulbactam, amoxicillin-clavulanic acid)

b) Penicillin Binding Protein (PBP): a mutation in the usual protein bound by penicillins makes *S. aureus* resistant to even methicillin/oxacillin/nafcillin (MRSA)

c) For many years MRSA was exclusively seen in the hospital (i.e., nosocomial), and was multi-drug resistant, requiring the use of vancomycin, however since approximately 2001–2002, there has been an explosion in community-acquired MRSA infections, and these isolates are often susceptible to older drugs, including trimethoprim-sulfamethoxazole, clindamycin, and doxycycline/minocycline

      d) Linezolid and daptomycin are newer agents that retain activity against virtually all strains of MRSA thus far

   8) Prophylaxis: strict contact isolation and hand-washing; for patients with recurrent *Staph.* infections (often MRSA), eradication of nasal carriage with mupirocin ointment can be attempted to decrease the frequency of recurrences

  b. *S. epidermidis*

   1) Appearance: GPC in clusters, colonies appear white on Petri dish

   2) Lab assays: **coagulase negative, novobiocin sensitive** (killed by novobiocin), catalase positive

   3) Virulence factors: mucopolysaccharide (slime) allowing adhesion to plastic surfaces

   4) Epidemiology: ubiquitous human skin flora

   5) Clinical Diseases:

     a) Bacteremia: **nosocomial infections via intravenous catheters**; often a contaminant from inadequate sterilization of skin prior to drawing the blood cultures

     b) Endocarditis: risk greatest for prosthetic valves within 6 months of valve replacement

     c) Prosthesis: bacteremia secondary to line infections can seed any plastic prosthetic

   6) Treatment: vancomycin frequently required, linezolid and daptomycin are newer options

   7) Resistance: intrinsically resistant to most antibiotics

   8) Prophylaxis: sterility during surgery and line placement

  c. *S. saprophyticus*

   1) Appearance: GPC in clusters, colonies appear white on Petri dish

   2) Lab assays: **coagulase negative, novobiocin resistant**, catalase positive

   3) Virulence factors: epithelial adhesins

   4) Epidemiology: genitourinary mucosa flora

   5) Clinical Diseases: outpatient urinary tract infection (UTI) in young women

   6) Treatment: trimethoprim-sulfamethoxazole or fluoroquinolones

   7) Resistance: intrinsically resistant to most penicillins

   8) Prophylaxis: none

2. *Streptococcus*

α-hemolytic *Streptococci*

- α = partial hemolysis

- Forms green zone around colonies on blood agar Petri dish due to partial degradation of red blood cells

TABLE 2.1	**Summary of *Staphylococcus* spp.**			
	APPEARANCE	**LAB**	**VIRULENCE**	**EPIDEM.**
aureus	GPC clusters; **Gold** colonies	**Coagulase** $\oplus$	Toxins	Colonizes skin
epidermidis	GPC clusters; White colonies	Coagulase –; Novobiocin sensitive	**Plastic** adhesins	Colonizes skin
saprophyticus	GPC clusters; White colonies	Coagulase –; **Novobiocin resistant**	Mucosal adhesins	Colonizes GU mucosa

a. *S. pneumonia*
  1) Appearance: **GPC in pairs** (also known as diplococci)
  2) Lab assays: **susceptible to bile, deoxycholate, and optochin, quellung reaction positive** (swelling of polysaccharide capsule in presence of immune serum), catalase negative (**all *streptococci* are catalase negative**)
  3) Virulence factors:
    a) IgA protease: degrades IgA in mucosal secretions
    b) Polysaccharide capsule: inhibits phagocytosis
  4) Epidemiology:
    a) Colonizes oropharynx in up to 50% of people
    b) Host factors are crucial to allowing infection: **splenectomy, HIV, malnutrition, alcoholism, chronic lung disease, nephrotic syndrome, multiple myeloma, or in general, anything that inhibits host antibody responses markedly increases host susceptibility to *S. pneumonia***
  5) Clinical Diseases:
    a) Pneumonia (**#1 cause of community acquired pneumonia**), often with bacteremia
    b) Meningitis (**#1 cause**)
    c) Otitis media/Sinusitis
    d) Bronchitis
  6) Treatment: penicillins, cephalosporins, macrolides, extended spectrum quinolones (e.g., levofloxacin/moxifloxacin/gatifloxacin)
  7) Resistance:
    a) Increasing resistance to penicillins due to altered Penicillin Binding Protein
    b) High level resistance to 3rd generation cephalosporins is rare but increasing
    c) Macrolide resistance, and even increasing quinolones resistance, tracks with penicillin resistance

8) Prophylaxis:
   a) Pneumovax is a polyvalent polysaccharide vaccine composed of capsular antigens from 23 *S. pneumonia* isotypes
   b) **Pneumovax should be given to all people ≥ 65 years old, all patients without spleens, and all patients with chronic debilitating illnesses** (e.g., heart failure, lung diseases, cirrhosis, renal failure, cancers, alcoholism, etc.)
   c) A conjugated protein-carrier vaccine with capsular antigens from seven isotypes is administered to children

b. Viridans group *Streptococci* (Viridans derives from the Latin word for "green," named for their α-hemolysis, refers to a number of different relatively avirulent Strep species)
   1) Appearance: GPC in chains
   2) Lab assays: **resistant to bile, deoxycholate, and optochin, quellung reaction negative**, catalase negative
   3) Virulence factors: none significant
   4) Epidemiology: human mouth flora
   5) Clinical Diseases: endocarditis, **keys to diagnosis are history of poor dentition or recent dental procedures**
   6) Treatment: penicillin + aminoglycoside, or 3rd generation cephalosporin
   7) Resistance: unusual
   8) Prophylaxis: ampicillin prior to dental procedures, good dentition

β-hemolytic *Streptococci*

- β = complete hemolysis, forms clear zone around colonies on blood agar Petri dish
- Lancefield system: a subclassification of β-hemolytic *Streptococci* based upon the C-carbohydrate in the organism's cell wall—only β-hemolytic Strep are classified by this system, so the terms Group A, Group B, or Group D Strep always refer to β-hemolytic Strep
- Groups C, E–G are rarely pathogenic and are not discussed

c. *S. pyogenes* (Group A Strep)
   1) Appearance: GPC in chains
   2) Lab assays: **bacitracin sensitive**, catalase negative
   3) Virulence factors:
      a) **M protein**: an anti-phagocytic component of the polysaccharide capsule, polymorphisms in the M protein allow subclassification of Group A Strep to identify individual strains—antibody to one form of M-protein provides immunity only to that particular strain of Group A Strep
      b) Streptolysin O causes β-hemolysis, immune response to it generates an antibody commonly assayed for to detect the presence of Group A Strep, called the **anti-streptolysin O (ASO) antibody**

    c) Exotoxin A & B: A is a superantigen, while B causes the tissue necrosis seen in necrotizing fasciitis

    d) **Erythrogenic toxin causes scarlet fever**

4) Epidemiology: frequently colonizes human skin, occasionally the oropharynx

5) Clinical Diseases:

    a) Pharyngitis—classic Strep throat, can progress to otitis/sinusitis

    b) Cellulitis/impetigo/erysipelas

    c) Necrotizing fasciitis: **the classic flesh-eating virus, which, ironically, is not a virus and does not "eat" the flesh** (it necrotizes tissue by secreting exotoxin B)

    d) Post-streptococcal glomerulonephritis: **immune complex deposition** causes rapidly progressive nephritic syndrome, although acute renal failure develops, it is typically self-limiting—note, this occurs 2–3 weeks after the resolution of any Strep infection (cellulitis, pharyngitis, or other)

    e) Rheumatic fever: due to an **immunologic cross-reaction (molecular mimicry)** with a Group A Strep antigen, resulting in heart valve damage, fever, rash, migratory polyarthritis, choreiform movements, with elevated ASO titers—the disease occurs 2 weeks after a Group A Strep infection, and can be prevented by antibiotic treatment within the first week of infection

    f) Scarlet fever: a self-limiting exfoliative disorder due to erythrogenic toxin, resulting in the classic sandpaper-like maculopapular eruption

6) Treatment: 100% of strains susceptible to penicillin

7) Resistance: none

8) Prophylaxis: antibiotic therapy prevents glomerulonephritis and rheumatic fever

d. *S. agalactiae* (Group B Strep)

1) Appearance: GPC in chains, occasionally in pairs

2) Lab assays: **bacitracin resistant, hydrolyzes hippurate, CAMP factor positive** (causes synergistic hemolysis with *S. aureus*), catalase negative

3) Virulence factors: an antiphagocytic capsule

4) Epidemiology:

    a) Colonizes female genitourinary tract

    b) **Group B Strep in the urine is a marker for high organism burden**

    c) **Prolonged rupture of membranes is the key risk factor to neonatal transmission**

    d) **Premature infants are at increased risk for infection**

5) Clinical Diseases: neonatal bacteremia and meningitis (it is the most common cause in neonates)

6) Treatment: penicillins +/– aminoglycoside

7) Resistance: none
8) Prophylaxis: treat pregnant women colonized with Group B Strep with ampicillin during labor, and treat women with prolonged rupture of membranes

e. *S. bovis* (Group D Strep)
1) Appearance: GPC in chains
2) Lab assays: **resistant to bile, hydrolyze esculin** (produce black pigment on bile/esculin agar), **susceptible to hypertonic saline** (note: this differentiates them from *Enterococcus*, which used to be classified as Group D Strep, see below), catalase negative
3) Virulence factors: none significant
4) Epidemiology: human intestinal flora
5) Clinical Diseases: bacteremia and endocarditis—note, up to 50% of patients with *S. bovis* endocarditis have an underlying colon cancer that allowed the organism to translocate into the bloodstream, **so always think colon cancer if this organism comes up on the boards**
6) Treatment: penicillins
7) Resistance: none
8) Prophylaxis: none

γ-hemolytic *Streptococci*

- γ = lack of hemolysis
- Strains from a number of species can be γ-hemolytic, including Viridans Strep (usually α-hemolytic), *S. bovis* (usually β-hemolytic), as well as *Enterococcus* (see below)

3. *Enterococci*
   a. *E. faecalis* & *E. faecium*
   1) Appearance: GPC in chains & pairs
   2) Lab assays: **resistant to bile, hydrolyze esculin** (produce black pigment on bile/esculin agar), **resistant to hypertonic saline** (this distinguishes them from *S. bovis*, which is susceptible to hypertonic saline)
   3) Virulence factors: none significant
   4) Epidemiology: human intestinal flora
   5) Clinical Diseases:
      a) UTI
      b) Biliary infections (e.g., cholangitis)
      c) Abdominal/pelvic abscesses
      d) Endocarditis
   6) Treatment:
      a) Vancomycin-susceptible *Enterococcus*: ampicillin is by far the most active antibiotic against *Enterococcus*, only if it is resistant or the patient is intolerant should other agents, such as vancomycin, possibly with aminoglycoside for synergy, be used

TABLE 2.2	Summary of *Streptococcus & Enterococcus spp.*			
	APPEARANCE	**LAB**	**VIRULENCE**	**EPIDEM.**
		Streptococcus spp.		
pneumonia	GPC **pairs**	α-hemolytic **quellung positive**	Capsule	**Splenectomy,** HIV+, alcohol, chronic disease
viridans	GPC chains	α-hemolytic **resistant to bile/optochin/ deoxycholate**	None	**Dental procedures cause infxn**
pyogenes	GPC chains	β-hemolytic **bacitracin sensitive**	**M Protein, streptolysin O**	Skin flora
agalactiae	GPC chains	β-hemolytic **bacitracin resistant, CAMP factor positive**	Capsule	Female GU tract, **neonatal infections**
bovis	GPC chains	β or γ- hemolytic, **resistant to bile, hydrolyzes esculin, inhibited by hypertonic saline**	None	Lives in colon, **colon cancer** predisposes to infection
		Enterococcus spp.		
faecalis/ faecium	GPC chains/ pairs	α, β, or γ- hemolytic, **resistant to bile, hydrolyzes esculin, resistant to hypertronic saline**	None	Intestinal flora, participates in polymicrobial infections

TABLE 2.3	**Laboratory Summary of Gram Positive Cocci**			
	APPEARANCE	**CATALASE**	**HEMOLYSIS**	**UNIQUE PROPERTY**
Staphylococcus spp.				
aureus	Clusters	⊕	β	Coagulase ⊕, gold colonies
epidermidis	Clusters	⊕	γ	Novobiocin sensitive
saprophyticus	Clusters	⊕	γ	Novobiocin resistant
Streptococcus spp.				
pneumonia	Pairs	—	α	Quellung reaction ⊕
Viridans	Chains	—	α, γ	Resist bile/ deoxycholate/ optochin
pyogenes	Chains	—	β	Bacitracin sensitive
agalactiae	Chains	—	β	Bacitracin resistant, CAMP ⊕
bovis	Chains	—	β or γ	Resist bile, lysed by hypertonic saline
Enterococcus spp.				
faecalis/faecium	Chains/pairs	—	α, β, or γ	Resist bile & hypertonic saline

       b) Vancomycin-Resistant Enterococcus (VRE): newer antibiotics, such as linezolid and daptomycin, are options

    7) Resistance: intrinsically resistant to most antibiotics, *faecium* spp. are particularly resistant

    8) Prophylaxis: hand-washing, contact isolation

B. Gram Positive Rods (GPR)

    1. *Bacillus*

       a. *B. anthracis*

          1) Appearance: GPR with square ends in a chain, **appear like box-cars on a train**

          2) Lab assays: **non-motile**, spore-forming anaerobe

3) Virulence factors:
 a) Anti-phagocytic capsule made of **D-glutamate**
 b) Anthrax toxin
  i) Tripartite toxin: protective antigen, lethal factor, and edema factor
  ii) Edema factor acts via adenylate cyclase
4) Epidemiology: spores in soil, or on animal hide, fur, or wool transmitted via epithelial penetration or inhalation
5) Clinical Diseases:
 a) Anthrax is a systemic sepsis syndrome characterized by a black eschar at the portal of entry, called a **"malignant pustule"**
 b) Woolsorter's disease is a severe pneumonic process caused by inhalation of spores, rapidly fatal—a classic early finding is a widened mediastinum on CXR, due to massive mediastinal lymphadenopathy
 c) From a bioterrorism perspective, think of anthrax in a patient, possibly young and otherwise healthy, with a flu-like illness that progresses rapidly and inexplicably to fulminant sepsis with acute respiratory distress syndrome, with a widened mediastinum on CXR
 d) Meningitis with gram positive rods is another manifestation of disease
6) Treatment: current guidelines are to start with ciprofloxacin and/or doxycycline, and to narrow to penicillin if the organism is shown to be susceptible
7) Resistance: none significant
8) Prophylaxis: a moderately efficacious vaccine is available for those at high risk (e.g., abattoir workers, tanners, etc.); in the context of bioterrorism, contacts with potential exposures to bioterrorism sources can receive 60 days of ciprofloxacin or doxycycline

b. *B. cereus*
1) Appearance: GPR with square ends in a chain, **appear like box-cars on a train**
2) Lab assays: **motile**
3) Virulence factors: exotoxins causing gastroenteritis (i.e., enterotoxin)
4) Epidemiology: spores that germinate when heated found on grains/rice
5) Clinical Diseases: gastroenteritis **classically occurs when fried rice is reheated, can occur either rapidly (within 4 hrs of consumption, easily confused with *S. aureus* gastroenteritis) or after an 18-hr incubation**
6) Treatment: symptomatic support
7) Resistance: none
8) Prophylaxis: none

2. *Clostridium*
   a. *C. botulinum*
      1) Appearance: GPR with subterminal spores
      2) Lab assays: spore-forming **anaerobe**, inoculation of affected food or serum from patient causes botulism in mice
      3) Virulence factors: botulinum toxin is preformed, inactivated by high heat-cooking, absorbed in gut, carried by bloodstream to nerve endings where it blocks the release of acetylcholine into the nerve synapse
      4) Epidemiology: spores in soil and on contaminated foods, often canned foods; also seen in drug users injecting black tar heroin (especially in California) or rarely from traumatic or surgical wound inoculation (so-called wound botulism)
      5) Clinical Diseases:
         a) Classic botulism: after ingestion of food contaminated by spores, causes classic **"descending paralysis" with significant bulbar effects** (e.g., diplopia, dysphagia, cranial neuropathy) ultimately causing respiratory collapse
         b) Wound botulism: caused by contamination of wound by spores, presentation the same as classic botulism
         c) Infant botulism: **classically seen after ingestion of honey**, disease usually not fatal in infants
      6) Treatment: botulism antitoxin, respiratory support, debridement of infected wounds
      7) Resistance: none
      8) Prophylaxis: properly storing and cooking food, discard swollen cans
   b. *C. difficile*
      1) Appearance: GPR
      2) Lab assays: C-diff toxin screen in stool, anaerobic, form spores
      3) Virulence factors: exotoxins cause pseudomembranous colitis, with watery/bloody diarrhea, exotoxin B ADP-ribosylates a GTP-binding protein called Rho
      4) Epidemiology: transmitted fecal-orally, colonizes GI tract in up to a third of hospitalized patients, selected for by use of clindamycin (high risk of C-diff), penicillins, cephalosporins (#1 cause since they are used so frequently), and others
      5) Clinical Diseases: severe gastroenteritis, with blood and mucous, can cause systemic toxicity, toxic megacolon, colonoscopy shows classic "pseudomembranes" in colon
      6) Treatment: withdraw causative antibiotic, treat with oral metronidazole (1st line), or with oral vancomycin if the organism is resistant to metronidazole
      7) Resistance: rare
      8) Prophylaxis: avoid antibiotics

    c. *C. perfringens*
1) Appearance: GPR, **thick**, brick-like
2) Lab assays: β-hemolytic, anaerobic, form spores
3) Virulence factors: α-toxin destroys cell membranes, other enzymes cause gas to form in tissues
4) Epidemiology: spores ubiquitous in soil, bacteria are also normal colonic and vaginal flora
5) Clinical Diseases:
    a) Gas gangrene: infects dirty wounds, classically causes **crepitance** due to subcutaneous gas, very high mortality rate from systemic shock
    b) Gastroenteritis: a self-limited infection from reheating food, **incubation period is 8–16 hrs**, diarrhea is prominent but vomiting is not
6) Treatment: surgical debridement is first-line, penicillin and clindamycin are adjunctive
7) Resistance: none
8) Prophylaxis: clean wounds

    d. *C. tetani*
1) Appearance: GPR, **thin**, with **terminal spores, appears like a drumstick or tennis racket**
2) Lab assays: anaerobic, form spores
3) Virulence factors: tetanus toxin is an exotoxin produced at the site of inoculation, carried by bloodstream to peripheral nerves, transported retrograde up the axon to the proximal synapse where it inhibits the release of inhibitory signals like glycine, thereby causing unopposed stimulation of the nerve
4) Epidemiology: spores ubiquitous in soil and dirty metal or glass
5) Clinical Diseases: infects dirty wounds, causing permanent neuromuscular stimulation, classic findings are lockjaw from inability to relax jaw muscles, and risus sardonicus (sardonic smile), death is ultimately secondary to respiratory failure
6) Treatment: tetanus antitoxin immunoglobulin
7) Resistance: none
8) Prophylaxis: vaccination with tetanus toxoid, a formaldehyde inactivated toxin, for particularly dirty wounds, both toxoid and immunoglobulin should be given concurrently

3. *Corynebacterium*
    a. *C. diphtheriae*
1) Appearance: GPR, thin, **club-shaped, arranged in palisades, V- or L-shaped formations, granules stain metachromatically** (granules stain different color than the rest of the cell)

TABLE 2.4	**Summary of Gram Positive Rods**			
	APPEARANCE	**LAB**	**VIRULENCE**	**EPIDEM.**
		Bacillus		
anthracis	In a chain, like box-cars	Non-motile, spore-forming anaerobe	D-glutamate capsule, tripartite toxin	Spores in soil, animal hide/ fur
cereus	In a chain, like box-cars	Motile, spore-forming anaerobe	Enterotoxin	**Reheated fried rice**
		Clostridium		
botulinum	Subterminal spore	Spore-forming anaerobe	Botulinum toxin blocks acetylcholine	Spores in soil and canned food
difficile	GPR	Anaerobe, C-diff toxin in stool	C-diff toxin	Antibiotics predispose
perfringens	Thick GPR	Anaerobic, spore forming	α-toxin	Spores in soil
tetani	Thin GPR, appears like a drumstick	Anaerobic, spore forming	Tetanus toxin	Spores in soil, dirty glass or metal
		Corynebacterium		
diphtheriae	Thin, palisades, metachromatic granules	Non-motile, aerobe, forms black colonies on tellurite agar: Schick's test discerns immunity or not	Diphtheria toxin	Respiratory droplets
		Listeria		
monocytogenes	Tumbling motility	Motile, aerobe, β-hemolytic	Listerio-lysin O	Unpasteurized dairy products

2) Lab assays: **non-motile**, not anaerobic (as opposed to *Clostridium*), do not form spores, **form black colonies on tellurite agar**; Schick's test is the injection of pure diphtheria toxin intradermally into a patient, if no inflammation occurs the patient is immune (historical interest only)
3) Virulence factors: diphtheria toxin ADP-ribosylates elongation factor 2 (EF-2), thereby inhibiting protein synthesis in the cell
4) Epidemiology: transmitted from the oropharynx by respiratory droplets
5) Clinical Diseases: diphtheria is typified by airway obstruction via formation of a **gray, fibrinous pseudomembrane in the oropharynx**, myocarditis can also develop
6) Treatment: antitoxin, respiratory support
7) Resistance: none
8) Prophylaxis: diphtheria toxoid, should be given to all children as part of the DTP vaccine

4. *Listeria*
   a. *L. monocytogenes*
      1) Appearance: GPR, thin, arranged in palisades, V- or L-shaped formations
      2) Lab assays: classic **tumbling motility**, not anaerobic, do not form spores, β-hemolytic
      3) Virulence factors: listeriolysin O disrupts cell membranes
      4) Epidemiology: transmitted via unpasteurized dairy products or via fecal-oral route
      5) Clinical Diseases:
         a) Neonatal meningitis or sepsis, abortion
         b) Bacteremia and meningitis occur in the immunocompromised, such as patients on corticosteroids, transplant patients, alcoholics, but also in pregnant women
      6) Treatment: ampicillin +/– aminoglycoside
      7) Resistance: unusual
      8) Prophylaxis: pasteurize cheese and dairy products

C. Gram Negative Cocci (GNC)

1. *Neisseria*
   a. *N. meningitidis*
      1) Appearance: **often diplococci**, arranged like **two kidney beans** facing each other
      2) Lab assays: grow on chocolate agar (heated blood agar), oxidase positive, ferments maltose
      3) Virulence factors:
         a) Antiphagocytic capsule
         b) IgA protease

4) Epidemiology: transmitted via respiratory droplets, colonize oropharynx, prone to outbreaks in communal settings such as college dormitory or military barracks, **people with defects in the late complement pathway (C6–C9) are prone to *Neisseria* infections**

5) Clinical Diseases:
   a) Meningitis
   b) Waterhouse–Friderichsen syndrome: sepsis resulting in DIC and adrenal failure due to adrenal gland infarction

6) Treatment: penicillin

7) Resistance: rare

8) Prophylaxis: a moderately efficacious vaccine is available for those at high risk (e.g., college freshmen in dormitories, those in military barracks, etc.), rifampin or fluoroquinolones are used for primary prophylaxis of close contacts of an infected patient

b. *N. gonorrhea*
   1) Appearance: often **diplococci inside neutrophils** (pathogno-monic on Gram stain from urethral specimen)
   2) Lab assays: **growth on Thayer–Martin agar** (chocolate agar with antibiotics to suppress genitourinary colonizers), oxidase positive, does not ferment maltose
   3) Virulence factors:
      a) Pili attach to mucosal surfaces
      b) Lipo-oligosaccharide (LOS) instead of lipopolysaccharide (LPS) makes the organism less stimulatory to immune cells
      c) IgA protease
   4) Epidemiology: always sexually transmitted, in both males and females infection can be asymptomatic, **infections common in patients with late complement deficiencies (C6–C9)**
   5) Clinical Diseases:
      a) Urethritis, pharyngitis, proctitis
      b) Pelvic inflammatory disease, salpingitis
      c) Septic arthritis
   6) Treatment: ceftriaxone, fluoroquinolones 2nd line
   7) Resistance: common to penicillins, due both to altered peni-cillin binding proteins and expression of β-lactamase
   8) Prophylaxis: safe sex

2. *Moraxella catarrhalis*
   1) Appearance: paired coccobacilli (rods are very short) often inside neutrophils
   2) Lab assays: oxidase positive, does not ferment maltose
   3) Virulence factors: none significant
   4) Epidemiology: respiratory droplet transmission, colonizes human oropharynx

TABLE 2.5	Summary of Gram Negative Cocci			
	APPEARANCE	**LAB**	**VIRULENCE**	**EPIDEM.**
N. meningitidis	Diplococci, often intracellular	Oxidase positive, ferments maltose	Capsule	Communal outbreaks
N. gonorrhea	Diplococci, often intracellular	Oxidase positive, does not ferment maltose, grows on Thayer-Martin media	Pili, LOS	STD, can be asymptomatic
M. catarrhalis	Paired coccobacillus (short rods)	Oxidase positive, does not ferment maltose	None sig.	Transmitted via respiratory droplets
Acinetobacter	Paired coccobacillus (medium rods)	Oxidase negative	None sig.	ICU colonizer, ventilator assoc. pneumonia

     5) Clinical Diseases:
        a) Upper respiratory diseases: otitis/sinusitis/bronchitis
        b) Atypical pneumonia
     6) Treatment: macrolide or doxycycline
     7) Resistance: frequent β-lactamase production
     8) Prophylaxis: none

  3. *Acinetobacter*
     1) Appearance: paired coccobacilli (rods are medium sized) often inside neutrophils
     2) Lab assays: oxidase negative
     3) Virulence factors: none significant
     4) Epidemiology: **transmission associated with pooled water, notorious ICU colonizer**
     5) Clinical Diseases:
        a) **Pneumonia: always nosocomial, usually in the ICU, often in patients on ventilators**
        b) Bacteremia, secondary to pneumonia
     6) Treatment: depends on susceptibility
     7) Resistance: **essentially 100% β-lactamase production, extremely resistant organism**, definitive therapy depends on particular sensitivity pattern of isolate
     8) Prophylaxis: contact isolation, ICU sterility

D. Gram Negative Rods (GNR)

1. Enterobacteriaceae

- A family of GNR, all are normal flora in the colon

- **All have four defining metabolic features: (1) facultative anaerobes, (2) ferment glucose, (3) oxidase negative, and (4) reduce nitrates to nitrites**

- Three classic antigens: (1) O antigen is a component of LPS in members of the Enterobacteriaceae, (2) H antigen is a flagellar protein found in *E. coli* and *Salmonella*, and (3) K antigen is a capsular polysaccharide antigen found in encapsulated organisms

- The genera are important, but individual species not important for exam purposes

  a. *Escherichia coli*

  1) Appearance: GNR

  2) Lab assays: **motile,** ferments lactose as detected by forming pink colonies on MacConkey agar and green colonies on EMB agar, forms gas but not hydrogen sulfide (H_2S) on triple sugar iron (TSI) agar, **metabolizes tryptophan to indole**

  3) Virulence factors:

     a) Pili allow mucosal adhesion

     b) Enterotoxins cause watery diarrhea

        i) Heat Stable Toxin (ST) ↑ cGMP levels in the cell, causing ion and fluid secretion

        ii) Heat Labile Toxin (LT) is almost identical to cholera toxin (see below), and ↑ cAMP

     c) **Shiga-toxin, found in *E. coli* O157:H7, causes bloody diarrhea and the hemolytic-uremic syndrome**

     d) Has O, H, and K antigens (see above)

     e) **LPS is a very potent stimulator of inflammation/sepsis**

  4) Epidemiology: normal colonic flora, gastroenteritis spread by fecal-oral contact

  5) Clinical Diseases:

     a) **Most common cause of UTI/pyelonephritis**

     b) Traveler's diarrhea (watery, non-bloody) caused by enterotoxigenic *E. coli* (ETEC)

     c) Dysentery/bloody gastroenteritis caused by enteroinvasive *E. coli* (EIEC)

     d) Hemolytic-uremic syndrome complicates gastroenteritis caused by enterohemorrhagic *E. coli* O157:H7 (EHEC), especially in children, presents with fulminant acute renal failure and sepsis-syndrome

     e) Neonatal meningitis

     f) Bacteremia causes classic gram negative sepsis

      6) Treatment: cephalosporins, trimethoprim-sulfamethoxazole, quinolones, aminoglycosides

      7) Resistance: increasing in the community to many antibiotics

      8) Prophylaxis: good hygiene

b. *Salmonella*

      1) Appearance: GNR

      2) Lab assays: **motile**, does not ferment lactose (clear colonies on MacConkey and EMB agar), produces gas and hydrogen sulfide on TSI agar

      3) Virulence factors:
         a) O, H, and K antigens
         b) *Salmonella* are subdivided by O antigens into groups A to I

      4) Epidemiology: **transmitted via poultry and eggs, gastric acid is crucial to host defense, so patients on acid-reduction therapy are prone to infection, can also be transmitted by pets such as turtles, lizards, and dogs**

      5) Clinical Diseases:
         a) Enterocolitis: bloody gastroenteritis, typically self-limited
         b) Typhoid fever: minimal GI symptoms, systemic dissemination causes fever with delirium and abdominal pain, **Rose spots** are classic rose-colored macules on the abdomen, some patients suffer intestinal perforation, during recovery *Salmonella* **colonizes the gallbladder readily and then is transmitted fecally in a carrier state (remember Typhoid Mary?)**
         c) Bacteremia: can seed any organ, frequently bone in asplenic patients (e.g., sickle cell), and can cause abdominal abscesses

      6) Treatment: cephalosporin, aminoglycoside, fluoroquinolone

      7) Resistance: unusual

      8) Prophylaxis: good hygiene

c. *Shigella*

      1) Appearance: GNR

      2) Lab assays: **non-motile**, does not ferment lactose (clear colonies on MacConkey and EMB agar), does not produce gas or hydrogen sulfide on TSI agar

      3) Virulence factors:
         a) O antigen only
         b) Some strains produce Shiga-toxin

      4) Epidemiology: transmitted via fecal-oral route and contaminated food, **only 100 organisms are required to establish enteric infection**

      5) Clinical Diseases: enterocolitis = bloody gastroenteritis, typically self-limited

      6) Treatment: supportive, fluids and electrolytes, fluoroquinolones or aminoglycosides for severe disease

       7) Resistance: increasing

       8) Prophylaxis: good hygiene

  d. *Yersinia enterocolitica* & *pseudotuberculosis* (see zoonotic infections for *Y. pestis*)

       1) Appearance: **oval shaped**

       2) Lab assays: **non-motile at 37°C but motile at 25°C**, do not ferment lactose, do not make gas or hydrogen sulfide on TSI agar, **urease positive**

       3) Virulence factors: enterotoxins

       4) Epidemiology: zoonotic transmission, fecal-oral

       5) Clinical Diseases:

          a) Gastroenteritis with bloody diarrhea, invasive disease

          b) **Mesenteric adenitis mimicking appendicitis**

       6) Treatment: trimethoprim-sulfamethoxazole or fluoro-quinolones

       7) Resistance: none

       8) Prophylaxis: none

  e. *Proteus*

       1) Appearance: GNR

       2) Lab assays: **motile/swarming**, does not ferment lactose, makes gas and hydrogen sulfide on TSI agar, **urease positive, phenylalanine deaminase positive**

       3) Virulence factors: urease splits urea, alkalinizing urine

       4) Epidemiology: causes community acquired UTIs and nosocomial infections

       5) Clinical Diseases:

          a) Community acquired or nosocomial UTIs

          b) **Causes infected struvite stones (ammonium magnesium phosphate) via alkalinization of the urine**

          c) Line sepsis

          d) Bacteremia/sepsis

       6) Treatment: 3rd generation cephalosporin, aminoglycoside, or fluoroquinolone

       7) Resistance: increasing resistance in nosocomial infections

       8) Prophylaxis: sterility during procedures and careful hand-washing

  f. *Klebsiella*

       1) Appearance: GNR

       2) Lab assays: **non-motile**, ferments lactose, makes gas but not hydrogen sulfide on TSI agar

       3) Virulence factors: large polysaccharide capsule (K antigen)

       4) Epidemiology: community acquired disease affects the elderly and immunocompromised (e.g., alcoholics, diabetics, etc.), but it is also a common nosocomial pathogen

    5) Clinical Diseases:
      a) UTI/pyelonephritis, commonly nosocomial
      b) Pneumonia, **classic "currant-jelly" sputum (thick blood), can progress to lung abscess, affects alcoholics, diabetics, and those with chronic lung disease**
      c) Bacteremia/sepsis
    6) Treatment: 3rd generation cephalosporin, aminoglycoside, or fluoroquinolone
    7) Resistance: increasing resistance in nosocomial infections
    8) Prophylaxis: sterility during procedures and careful hand-washing

g. *Enterobacter*
    1) Appearance: GNR
    2) Lab assays: **motile**, ferments lactose, makes gas but not hydrogen sulfide on TSI agar
    3) Virulence factors: none significant
    4) Epidemiology: **causes nosocomial infections**
    5) Clinical Diseases:
      a) Line sepsis
      b) UTI if catheter in place
      c) Bacteremia/sepsis
      d) Cholangitis
    6) Treatment: piperacillin-tazobactam, aminoglycoside or fluoro-quinolone or both, not ceftazidime due to extended spectrum β-lactamases (see below)
    7) Resistance: **expresses extended spectrum β-lactamases (ESBL), making it resistant to all penicillin-derivatives (may be reversed with β-lactamase inhibitor, i.e., tazobactam), including ceftazidime**
    8) Prophylaxis: sterility during procedures and careful hand-washing

h. *Serratia*
    1) Appearance: GNR
    2) Lab assays: **motile**, does not ferment lactose, does not make gas or hydrogen sulfide on TSI agar
    3) Virulence factors: none significant
    4) Epidemiology: **causes nosocomial infections**
    5) Clinical Diseases:
      a) Line sepsis
      b) UTI if catheter in place
      c) Bacteremia/sepsis
    6) Treatment: 3rd generation cephalosporin, aminoglycoside, or fluoroquinolone
    7) Resistance: increasing resistance in nosocomial infections
    8) Prophylaxis: sterility during procedures and careful hand-washing

TABLE 2.6	**Summary of Enterobacteriaceae**				
	MOTILE	**FERMENTS LACTOSE**	**TSI AGAR: GAS/H₂S**	**UNIQUE CHARACTERISTIC**	**CAUSES ENTERITIS?**
E. coli	Yes	Yes	+/–	Metabolize tryptophan to indole	Yes
Salmonella	Yes	No	+/+	Colonize gallbladder	Yes
Shigella	No	No	–/–	Inoculum of 100 causes disease	Yes
*Yersinia spp.**	Yes†	No	–/–	Urease ⊕	Yes
Proteus	Yes	No	+/+	Swarming motility, urease & phenylalanine deaminase ⊕	No
Klebsiella	No	Yes	+/–	Large polysaccharide capsule	No
Enterobacter	Yes	Yes	+/–	Nosocomial pathogen	No
Serratia	Yes	No	–/–	Nosocomial pathogen	No

* *Y. enterocolitica* & *pseudotuberculosis* only, see Table 2.9 for *Y. pestis*.
† Mobile at 25°C but not 37°C.

2. Other GNR causing enteric infections

   a. *Vibrio cholera*

     1) Appearance: GNR, **shaped like a comma (curved)**

     2) Lab assays: motile, oxidase positive, **inhibited by hypertonic saline**

     3) Virulence factors: Enterotoxin composed of two subunits, A and B

       a) Subunit A ADP-ribosylates G-protein, locking it in the stimulatory mode, resulting in overwhelming production of cAMP → secretion of chloride ion and water in the small intestine

       b) Subunit B is necessary for penetration of Subunit A into the cell

     4) Epidemiology: Fecal-oral transmission, can also be transmitted via uncooked shellfish, carriers can be asymptomatic

5) Clinical Diseases:
   a) Watery diarrhea known as "rice–water stool," no blood in the diarrhea and no abdominal pain, death is due to dehydration and electrolyte imbalance; diarrhea is secretory, originates in the small intestine
6) Treatment: **oral rehydration with salt solution, glucose must be included in the rehydration solution to increase ion uptake in the gut via the sodium–glucose cotransporter;** antibiotics not indicated
7) Resistance: none
8) Prophylaxis: good hygiene and public health efforts

b. *Vibrio parahaemolyticus*
   1) Appearance: GNR, **shaped like a comma (curved)**
   2) Lab assays: motile, oxidase positive, **resistant to hypertonic saline**
   3) Virulence factors: Enterotoxin similar to *V. cholera*
   4) Epidemiology: **The bacteria lives in the ocean, typically transmitted by uncooked fish** (common cause of diarrhea in Japan and on cruise ships)
   5) Clinical Diseases: diarrhea of variable severity, typically self-limited, diarrhea is caused by enteroinvasion of colon and can sometimes be bloody
   6) Treatment: supportive
   7) Resistance: none
   8) Prophylaxis: adequately cooking seafood

c. *Vibrio vulnificus*
   1) Appearance: GNR, **shaped like a comma (curved)**
   2) Lab assays: motile, oxidase positive, **resistant to hypertonic saline**
   3) Virulence factors: none significant
   4) Epidemiology: Like *V. parahaemolyticus*, ***V. vulnificus* also lives in the ocean, typically transmitted via contact with fresh shellfish**
   5) Clinical Diseases:
      a) **Cellulitis in fishermen/shellfish handlers**
      b) **Severe sepsis in patients with cirrhosis** or other chronic diseases who ingest raw shellfish infected with the organism
   6) Treatment: 3rd generation cephalosporin +/– doxycycline or fluoroquinolone
   7) Resistance: poorly characterized
   8) Prophylaxis: adequately cooking seafood

d. *Campylobacter jejuni*
   1) Appearance: GNR, **shaped like an "S"**
   2) Lab assays: motile, oxidase positive, **microaerophilic** (grows better in 5% O_2 than 20%), urease negative
   3) Virulence factors: can produce a cholera-like toxin

    4) Epidemiology: Fecal-oral transmission, transmitted via domes-
ticated animals

    5) Clinical Diseases: **most common cause of bacterial gastroen-
teritis in the US**, the organism is invasive so blood and
mucous are typically found in the stool

    6) Treatment: 3rd generation cephalosporin or fluoro-
quinolone

    7) Resistance: increasing, even to quinolones

    8) Prophylaxis: adequately cooking seafood

e. *Helicobacter pylori*

    1) Appearance: GNR, **shaped like an "S"**

    2) Lab assays: motile, oxidase positive, **urease positive**

    3) Virulence factors: urease

    4) Epidemiology: Likely fecal-oral transmission

    5) Clinical Diseases: gastric/duodenal ulcers, gastric carcinoma
and lymphoma are associated with *H. pylori,* and **treating
H. pylori can make some lymphomas regress**

    6) Treatment: Triple Tx = amoxicillin + clarithromycin + omeprazole
(other regimens available as well)

    7) Resistance: increasing

    8) Prophylaxis: none

f. *Bacteroides fragilis*

    1) Appearance: GNR

    2) Lab assays: **strict anaerobe, non-spore forming**

    3) Virulence factors: antiphagocytic polysaccharide capsule

    4) Epidemiology: **most common bacteria in the intestines**, about
10^{11} per gram of feces, infections are all endogenous due to

TABLE 2.7	Summary of Enteric GNR		
	SHAPE	**LAB**	**HABITAT**
Vibrio cholera	Comma	Inhibited by hypertonic saline	Human host
Vibrio parahaemolyticus	Comma	**Resistant to hypertonic saline**	Ocean
Vibrio vulnificus	Comma	**Resistant to hypertonic saline**	Ocean
Campylobacter jejuni	Like an "S"	Microaerophilic, urease negative	Human host
Helicobacter pylori	Like an "S"	**Urease positive**	Human host
Bacteroides fragilis	GNR	**Strict anaerobe**	Human colon

translocation of *Bacteroides* across a break in the intestinal mucosa

5) Clinical Diseases: participates in polymicrobial abscesses, peritonitis, and sepsis following disruption of bowel

6) Treatment: metronidazole or a variety of 2nd line options (i.e., clindamycin, cefotetan, piperacillin/tazobactam, etc.)

7) Resistance: very rare to metronidazole, express β-lactamase

8) Prophylaxis: none

3. GNR causing respiratory infections
   a. *Hemophilus influenza*
      1) Appearance: cocco-bacillus (can be confused with cocci)
      2) Lab assays: Growth on chocolate agar requires supplementation with **Factor V (NAD) and Factor X (heme), quellung reaction positive**
      3) Virulence factors:
         a) Polysaccharide capsule allows identification of six serotypes, **of which type b is the most virulent due to its unique polyribitol phosphate capsule structure**
         b) IgA protease
      4) Epidemiology: Respiratory transmission, used to be the most common cause of meningitis but now is rare due to childhood vaccination
      5) Clinical Diseases:
         a) Community acquired pneumonia
         b) Bronchitis/sinusitis/otitis media
         c) Meningitis: **95% due to serotype b**, usually occurs between ages of 6 months to 2 years, after maternal IgG levels decline and before endogenous antibody is produced against the capsule
         d) In small children epiglottitis can occur, which is a medical emergency due to risk of laryngospasm causing respiratory arrest, presents with quiet/still child leaning forward and drooling due to inability to swallow, has classic "thumb" sign on lateral neck x-rays
      6) Treatment: meningitis requires 3rd generation cephalosporin, treat upper respiratory infections with amoxicillin or trimethoprim-sulfamethoxazole, treat pneumonia with 3rd generation cephalosporins or macrolides
      7) Resistance: many strains produce β-lactamase
      8) Prophylaxis:
         a) Extremely effective vaccine—**due to inability of small children to make specific antibodies directed at polysaccharide, the vaccine is a fusion of *H. influenza* polysaccharide linked to a carrier protein**
         b) Use rifampin for close contact prophylaxis for patients with meningitis

b. *Legionella pneumophila*
   1) Appearance: Gram stains faintly, hard to see
   2) Lab assays: **classically, sputum Gram stain shows neutrophils but no bacteria** (because they stain poorly), **require iron and cysteine supplementation to grow in culture**
   3) Virulence factors: none significant
   4) Epidemiology: Infectious outbreaks **associated with contaminated sources of water** (e.g., air conditioners, sinks, showers), although infections are transmitted via the lung, **person-to-person spread does not occur, most patients with severe disease are elderly, smoke, drink, or have a cell-mediated immune defect** (e.g., HIV, treated with steroids, renal transplant)
   5) Clinical Diseases:
      a) Pontiac fever: mild flu-like illness
      b) Severe multilobar pneumonia with systemic toxicity, **commonly associated with diarrhea** (always think *Legionella* in a patient with pneumonia and diarrhea), **very high LDH, pulse-fever dissociation, and hyponatremia**
   6) Treatment: 2nd generation macrolide (e.g., clarithromycin or azithromycin) and fluoroquinolones are both first line
   7) Resistance: frequently produce β-lactamases
   8) Prophylaxis: avoid contaminated water
c. *Bordetella pertussis*
   1) Appearance: small cocco-bacillus
   2) Lab assays: Growth requires **Bordet-Gengou agar**
   3) Virulence factors:
      a) Pili allow attachment to respiratory epithelia
      b) Pertussis toxin: **ADP-ribosylates an inhibitory G-protein**, blocking its activity, thereby allowing unopposed stimulation of adenylate cyclase → **high cAMP production** (contrast this with cholera toxin, which also stimulates high cAMP production but does so by ADP-ribosylating a stimulatory G-protein, thereby locking it into active form)
   4) Epidemiology: Highly contagious, transmitted by respiratory droplets, severe disease is rare in the developed world due to widespread vaccination, but it can cause chronic cough in adults
   5) Clinical Diseases:
      a) **Whooping cough: tracheobronchitis** affecting children, begins with a week of mild respiratory symptoms, followed by paroxysmal coughing attacks lasting up to 4 weeks (**the "whoop" is the characteristic sound made during the gasp for inhalation after a spasm of coughing**), pronounced lymphocytosis can occur
      b) A flu-like illness or chronic cough can occur in adults whose immunity has waned

6) Treatment: supportive, macrolides to shorten duration
7) Resistance: none
8) Prophylaxis: both whole cell, killed vaccine (part of DTP) and an acellular vaccine are in widespread use

d. *Pseudomonas aeruginosa*
1) Appearance: GNR
2) Lab assays: strict aerobe, oxidase positive, does not ferment glucose (in contrast to Enterobacteriaceae), does not ferment lactose (clear colonies on MacConkey or EMB agar), secretes pyocyanin and pyoverdin, which cause agar to become blue-green colored around a colony, **causes a fruity smell**, does not form gas or H_2S on TSI agar
3) Virulence factors:
   a) Glycocalyx slime prevents phagocytosis
   b) Exotoxin A works like diphtheria toxin, ADP-ribosylates EF-2, preventing protein synthesis
4) Epidemiology: common environmental water colonizer, rarely colonizes human colon, is fastidious and can survive disinfectants, as a result **is a major nosocomial pathogen**
5) Clinical Diseases:
   a) **Nosocomial infections**: UTI, pneumonia, bacteremia
   b) Commonly infects burns or open wounds
   c) Hot-tub cellulitis
   d) **Malignant otitis externa in diabetics**
   e) **Recurrent pneumonia in cystic fibrosis patients**
6) Treatment: **double cover** with a combination of ceftazidime, extended spectrum penicillin with β-lactamase inhibitor (e.g., piperacillin/tazobactam), aminoglycoside, or ciprofloxacin

TABLE 2.8	Summary of Respiratory GNR	
ORGANISM	**LAB**	**INFECTIONS**
Hemophilus	Factor V (NAD) & Factor X (heme) required for growth, quellung reaction ⊕	Rare now due to vaccine
Legionella	Iron & cysteine required for growth, Gram stain shows multiple neutrophils but no bacteria (stain poorly)	Water is the source; diarrhea, ↑ LDH, pulse-fever dissociation, & hyponatremia commonly seen
Bordetella	Grow on Bordet-Gengou agar	Very contagious
Pseudomonas	Agar turns green due to pyocyanin & pyoverdin, causes a fruity smell	Nosocomial pathogen, highly antibiotic resistant

7) Resistance: highly resistant to multiple antibiotics, and new **resistance occurs quickly on single therapy, so often double cover for severe disease**

8) Prophylaxis: hand-washing, sterility during procedures

4. GNR causing zoonotic infections

    a. *Bartonella henselae* & *quintana*

      1) Appearance: small coccobacillus

      2) Lab assays: diagnosis made by serology or biopsy

      3) Virulence factors: none significant

      4) Epidemiology: **body louse is proven to transmit *B. quintana*, *B. henselae* can be transmitted by cat scratches (particularly kittens)** and also possibly by body louse or fleas, *B. quintana* is associated with poor sanitation and cramped conditions such as refugee camps or trenches during war, while *B. henselae* is associated with homelessness

      5) Clinical Diseases:

        a) Cat-scratch disease: caused by *B. henselae*, presents with constitutional symptoms (e.g., fevers, chills, night-sweats), and diffuse, **massive lymphadenopathy affecting nodes nearest inoculation** (e.g., if scratch is on forearm nodes, extend up the arm to the axilla), can mimic lymphoma

        b) Bacillary angiomatosis: also caused by *B. henselae*, **a disseminated disease typically seen in AIDS patients**, bacteremia with fevers, chills, myalgias, and **characteristic red nodules all over the body** composed of **small capillary hemangiomas** which can appear like Kaposi's sarcoma

        c) Trench fever: caused by *B. quintana*, transmitted by body louse, presents with abrupt onset high fevers, chills, myalgias, can cause multiple paroxysms of fever separated by afebrile periods

      6) Treatment: doxycycline, macrolides, or fluoroquinolones

      7) Resistance: none

      8) Prophylaxis: good hygiene, avoid scratches by kittens

    b. *Brucella*

      1) Appearance: small coccobacillus

      2) Lab assays: diagnosis made by serology

      3) Virulence factors: none significant

      4) Epidemiology: **transmitted via unpasteurized contaminated milk or via direct contact with sheep, pigs, or cattle**

      5) Clinical Diseases:

        a) **Undulating fever: mono-like illness with constitutional symptoms, hepatosplenomegaly and diffuse adenopathy, fever waxes and wanes daily**

        b) Other manifestations include osteomyelitis (often of the spine, can appear like TB), meningitis, endocarditis, etc.

      6) Treatment: doxycycline plus aminoglycoside

      7) Resistance: rare

      8) Prophylaxis: pasteurize milk

  c. *Francisella tularensis*

      1) Appearance: small coccobacillus

      2) Lab assays: not cultured in lab due to risk of inhalational infection, diagnosis made by DFA or agglutination

      3) Virulence factors: none significant

      4) Epidemiology: typical host is rabbit or vermin, **usually transmitted by tick (also by lice or mite)**

      5) Clinical Diseases:

         a) Multiple forms of disease, most common is "ulceroglandular" type, an ulceration occurs at the site of inoculation, and diffuse lymphadenopathy develops, causing mono-like illness, can also cause pneumonia, and fulminant sepsis

         b) Disease typically from ticks acquired on the east coast, but also considered a potential bioterrorism pathogen

      6) Treatment: aminoglycoside

      7) Resistance: none

      8) Prophylaxis: live attenuated vaccine, moderately effective, given to people whose occupation places them at high risk (e.g., tanner, fur-trapper)

  d. *Pasteurella multocida*

      1) Appearance: small coccobacillus, **bipolar staining** (like a safety pin, the ends stain but clear in the middle)

      2) Lab assays: none helpful, diagnosis is presumptive/clinical

      3) Virulence factors: antiphagocytic capsule

      4) Epidemiology: **inoculated during dog or cat bites**, part of a polymicrobial cellulitis

      5) Clinical Diseases: **dog- or cat-bite cellulitis**

      6) Treatment: amoxicillin/clavulonic acid for polymicrobial infection

      7) Resistance: β lactamase causes penicillin resistance

      8) Prophylaxis: animal bites should not be sutured to prevent abscess formation

  e. *Yersinia pestis*

      1) Appearance: small coccobacillus, **bipolar staining** (like a safety pin, the ends stain but clear in the middle)

      2) Lab assays: great care must be taken during culturing to prevent airborne infection in the lab

      3) Virulence factors: antiphagocytic capsule

      4) Epidemiology: majority of cases in the world occur in SE Asia, but plague is endemic in the western U.S., host is vermin, vector is flea, person-to-person transmission also occurs via respiratory droplets

TABLE 2.9	Summary of Zoonotic GNR	
ORGANISM	**DISEASE CHARACTERISTICS**	**EPIDEMIOLOGY**
Bartonella henselae	Cat-scratch dz causes lymphadenopathy	Cat-scratch transmitted by kittens
	Bacillary angiomatosis causes diffuse skin hemangiomas	Bacillary angiomatosis typically seen in AIDS patients
Bartonella quintana	Trench fever with abrupt onset fever, can be paroxysmal	Seen in crowded, unsanitary conditions, associated with war and homelessness
Brucella	Undulating fever = waxes and wanes over weeks to months	Transmitted via dairy products, or contact with sheep, pigs, or cattle
Francisella	Ulceroglandular = ulcer forms at site of inoculation, diffuse adenopathy	Rabbit or vermin are host, vector is tick
Pasteurella	Cellulitis from dog or cat bites	Presumptive from dog or cat bites
Yersinia pestis	Buboes and rapid sepsis	Vermin are hosts, flea is vector

5) Clinical Diseases:
    a) Bubonic plague: **painful swelling of lymph nodes known as bubo typifies disease**, eventually the bubo ulcerates, within days the disease progresses to systemic toxicity, including severe pneumonia, DIC, sepsis/shock, **50% lethal without treatment**
    b) Pneumonic plague: **inhalation of contaminated respiratory droplets, much more rapid systemic course, 100% lethal without treatment**
6) Treatment: high dose gentamicin, treat preemptively, do NOT wait for Gram stain or culture results
7) Resistance: none
8) Prophylaxis: vermin control, flea control, quarantine infected patients

E. Atypical Bacteria (Gram Stain Unrevealing)

1. Acid Fast Bacteria
    a. *Mycobacterium avium-intracellulare*
       1) Appearance: acid fast bacilli
       2) Lab assays: cultures require up to 3 weeks to grow

3) Virulence factors: none significant
4) Epidemiology: ubiquitous in the environment, **disease develops in AIDS patients when CD4 count drops below 50**
5) Clinical Diseases:
   a) Disseminated disease: more common than pulmonary disease, causes fevers, weight loss, **lymphadenopathy, bone marrow suppression** (pancytopenia), and chronic gastroenteritis, seen when CD4 is less than 50
   b) Pulmonary disease: relatively rare, indistinguishable from TB clinically, classically NOT seen in HIV patients, but rather in patients with structural lung disease, and specifically in middle-aged/elderly Caucasian females with kyphosis/scoliosis with lingular or right middle lobe disease (the so-called Lady Windemere syndrome)
6) Treatment: multiple drug regimen, always include 2nd generation macrolide (clarithromycin or azithromycin) as cornerstone, rifampin/rifabutin, and ethambutol
7) Resistance: uncommon
8) Prophylaxis: all AIDS patients with CD4 counts less than 50 should receive azithromycin prophylaxis once per week

b. *Mycobacterium leprae*
   1) Appearance: acid fast bacilli seen within **foamy macrophages** (lipid laden) on biopsy
   2) Lab assays: obligate aerobe, cannot grow in culture, **must grow in armadillo footpads**, prefers growth at 30°C
   3) Virulence factors: none significant
   4) Epidemiology: transmitted by **prolonged** contact with secretions or skin of infected person, or possibly via contact with armadillos
   5) Clinical Diseases:
      a) **Lepromatous leprosy: the disseminated form seen in patients with poor cell-mediated immune responses to the organism,** the bacteria disseminates and grows uncontrolled in peripheral nerve endings, fingers, and earlobes (sites where body temperature is lower than core temperature)
      b) **Tuberculoid leprosy: strong delayed type hypersensitivity consistent with potent cell-mediated immunity, typified by relative control of disease with diminished organism burden on biopsy**
   6) Treatment: dapsone plus rifampin for up to 2 years
   7) Resistance: prone to resistance without dual therapy
   8) Prophylaxis: consider dapsone for close contacts

c. *Mycobacterium marinum*
   1) Appearance: acid fast bacilli
   2) Lab assays: **photochromogenic = forms yellow pigment when exposed to light**

3) Virulence factors: none significant
4) Epidemiology: lives in fresh water (e.g., fish tank, swimming pool)
5) Clinical Diseases: **"Fish-tank granuloma," infection develops after minor trauma causes break in skin with subsequent exposure of skin to fresh water environments,** results in progressive ulceration with heaped up borders
6) Treatment: 2nd generation macrolide (clarithromycin or azithromycin) or doxycycline
7) Resistance: none
8) Prophylaxis: avoid skin breaks

d. *Mycobacterium tuberculosis*
1) Appearance: cords of **acid fast bacilli,** stain red on Ziehl-Neelsen prep due to high cell wall content of mycolic acids
2) Lab assays: obligate aerobe, requires Lowenstein-Jensen medium for growth, doubling time = 18 hours (versus 20 minutes for *E. coli*) **so can take up to 8 weeks for cultures to grow, TB is the only *Mycobacterium* that produces niacin**
3) Virulence factors: cord factor allows growth in extended chains
4) Epidemiology: exposure is by respiratory droplets; however, **only 3% of exposed patients develop active disease per year, risk of active disease is increased by depressed immune status** (e.g., elderly, HIV+, malnourished, etc.)
5) Clinical Diseases:
   a) Pulmonary TB: **primary disease occurs in the lung bases, reactivation disease occurs in the upper lobes** due to higher oxygen tension which supports the organism better, disease course typified by chronic cough, hemoptysis, fevers, night sweats, weight loss, lymphadenopathy—**look for Ghon complex on CXR,** which is a granuloma with an adjacent calcified lymph node
   b) TB can disseminate to any organ
6) Treatment: four drug therapy = RIPE (rifampin, isoniazid, pyrazinamide, ethambutol) × 2 months, subsequently narrow to 2 drug therapy (isoniazid, rifampin) for a total of 6 months to 1 year of treatment
7) Resistance: increasingly common, multi-drug resistant (MDR) TB is of particular concern
8) Prophylaxis: based upon PPD test
   a) Purified Protein Derivative, administered intradermally, **useful as a screening test in asymptomatic patients but is NOT useful as a diagnostic test in symptomatic patients**
   b) Guidelines from 2000 recommend to prophylax all people with positive PPD regardless of age but to only put PPDs on people whom it is safe to prophylax (e.g., don't put a PPD on a low risk person >35 yrs old)

   i)   15 mm is positive in a healthy, asymptomatic person
        without risk of exposure
   ii) 10 mm is positive in an asymptomatic patient **with
        risks**, including **immigrant** from a high risk area (e.g.,
        SE Asia, Central/South America), pt from a medically
        underserved population (e.g., **homeless**), pt with a his-
        tory of recent **imprisonment**, pt **exposed to high risk
        individuals** (e.g., **health care workers** like us, **immigra-
        tion officers**, etc.)
   iii) 5 mm is positive in "high risk" pts, such as asymptom-
        atic pt with **known exposure** to someone with active
        disease or pt with **debilitating illness**, including **HIV,
        malignancy** of any kind, **cirrhosis, renal failure**, etc., or
        with CXR consistent with old disease
   iv) One-third of people with active pulmonary disease
        have negative PPDs with positive control (specifically
        anergic to TB) and 50% of people with disseminated
        disease have negative PPDs with positive control—
        **therefore PPD should NOT be used as a diagnostic test
        in someone with symptoms of active disease**
   c) **Prophylax all patients for 9 months regardless of HIV
      status (guidelines from 2000)**
   d) BCG vaccine is a live attenuated strain of *M. bovis* which
      shows some cross-protection to TB, but due to modest
      efficacy, short duration of protection, and invariable
      false-positive PPD seen after vaccination, it is not used
      in the U.S.
 e. *Nocardia*
   1) Appearance: thin **filaments or rods, acid fast and do not
      Gram stain** (see Figure 2.1)
   2) Lab assays: **aerobic, can cause an eosinophilia**
   3) Virulence factors: none significant
   4) Epidemiology: ubiquitous in environment, causes disease in
      immunocompromised
   5) Clinical Diseases: typically starts as pneumonia, but can
      disseminate especially to brain or kidneys, **mimics TB**
   6) Treatment: trimethoprim-sulfamethoxazole and surgical
      debridement
   7) Resistance: occasional
   8) Prophylaxis: none

2. Poorly Stained Bacteria
 a. *Actinomyces*
   1) Appearance: long, **filamentous** bacteria, **weakly gram
      positive**—NOT acid fast, distinguishes them from *Nocardia*
   2) Lab assays: anaerobic (also distinguishes from *Nocardia*, which is
      aerobic), **"sulfur granules"** are yellowish crystalloid-appearing

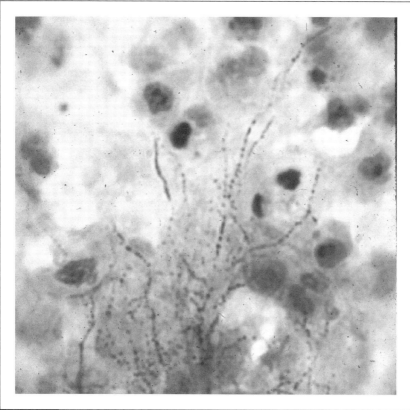

FIGURE 2.1 Microscopic Appearance of *Nocardia*

The typical microscopic appearance of Nocardia *in tissue, with long, thin, beaded, filamentous-like structures. Actinomyces appears similarly.*

clumps that are revealed to be clumped organisms when seen under microscope

3) Virulence factors: none significant

4) Epidemiology: normal flora of human oropharynx

5) Clinical Diseases: can cause abscesses and invasive infections in any organ, typically seen in head and neck, chest, or abdomen, dental infections common, **readily crosses tissue planes and erodes through bones, causing sinus tracts that drain from organs through the skin—"sinus tract" and "sulfur granules" are the key words to look for on an exam**

6) Treatment: penicillin and surgical debridement

7) Resistance: none

8) Prophylaxis: none

TABLE 2.10	Summary of Acid Fast Bacilli	
ORGANISM	**APPEARANCE**	**DISEASE CHARACTERISTICS**
M. avium intracellulare	Indistinguishable from TB by microscopy	Suspect in AIDS or cancer patient with pancytopenia and lymphadenopathy
M. leprae	AFBs in foamy macrophages	Organism grows in cool spots of body (e.g., ear lobes, nose, fingers, peripheral nerves)
M. marinum	Forms yellow pigment when exposed to light	"Fish-tank" granuloma, occurs following skin break and fresh water exposure
M. tuberculosis	AFBs in cords (chains)	Primary lung disease at bases, reactivation occurs at apices, look for Ghon complex = granuloma + calcified lymph node on CXR
Nocardia	Filamentous, weakly acid fast, variably Gram stains	Lung & brain infection in immunocompromised (e.g., steroids)

    b. *Chlamydia spp.*
        1) Appearance: form intracellular inclusion bodies, cannot be seen outside host cell
        2) Lab assays: all are obligate intracellular parasites, and cannot be grown on media, have complex life cycle including extracellular elementary body which is like a spore, and the intracellular reticulate body which is like a germinative form which undergoes fission to produce daughter elementary bodies, **seen as inclusion bodies inside cell**
        3) Virulence factors: none significant
        4) Epidemiology: *C. pneumonia* transmitted via respiratory droplets, *C. psittaci* transmitted via inhalation of bird feces, *C. trachomatis* transmitted via sexual contact or vertically at birth, and causes eye disease by direct finger/fomite to eye contact
        5) Clinical Diseases:
           a) *C. pneumonia*
              i)   Upper respiratory infections: otitis, sinusitis, bronchitis
              ii) Atypical pneumonia: nagging, non-productive, cough
           b) *C. psittaci* causes Psittacosis, pneumonia, high fever, headache
           c) *C. trachomatis*
              i)   Serotypes A–C cause **trachoma**: chronic conjunctivitis leading to scarring blindness over years, **this is the**

second most common cause of blindness worldwide
(behind cataracts)

  ii) Serotypes D–K cause GU infections: urethritis, prosta-
titis, cervicitis, pelvic inflammatory disease

  iii) Serotypes L1–L3 cause **lymphogranuloma venereum**: STD
with large inguinal adenopathy causing the **groove
sign** = groove of skin between two swollen lymph nodes

6) Treatment: macrolides or doxycycline, fluoroquinolones

7) Resistance: none

8) Prophylaxis: personal hygiene, safe sex

c. *Coxiella burnetii*

1) Appearance: can't be seen by light microscopy

2) Lab assays: obligate intracellular parasite, diagnosed by serology

3) Virulence factors: none significant

4) Epidemiology: transmitted via aerosolized particulates **from
exposure to farm animals like cattle, sheep, and goats, especially to products of conception (e.g., placenta)**

5) Clinical Diseases: Q fever = flu-like illness with fever and **particularly intense headache, and a classic combination of
pneumonia and hepatitis**, rash is distinctly unusual

6) Treatment: doxycycline

7) Resistance: none

8) Prophylaxis: avoid products of conception of farm animals

d. *Ehrlichia chaffeensis* & *Anaplasma phagocytophila*

1) Appearance: seen as intracellular inclusions in granulocytes
(*Anaplasma* = human granulocytic ehrlichiosis) or monocytes
(*Ehrlichia* = human monocytic ehrlichiosis)

2) Lab assays: serologies

3) Virulence factors: none significant

4) Epidemiology: transmitted by ticks in rural areas in the south
and east coast of the U.S.

5) Clinical Diseases:

  a) Human granulocytic ehrlichiosis and human monocytic
ehrlichiosis have similar presentations, with fevers, chills,
myalgias, occasional maculopapular rash, and a classic triad
of leukopenia, thrombocytopenia, and transaminitis, CNS
disease can occur

6) Treatment: doxycycline

7) Resistance: none

8) Prophylaxis: avoid tick exposures

e. *Mycoplasma pneumonia*

1) Appearance: Smallest bacteria, 0.3 μm in diameter, **lack cell
walls so cannot be seen on Gram stain**, in culture colonies
take on classic **"fried egg"** appearance with thick center and
flatter circular edge

2) Lab assays: must culture on media containing cholesterol because **Mycoplasma are the only bacteria that contain cholesterol in their cell membrane; cold agglutinins** are IgM antibodies which form against the organism, and cause red blood cell agglutination, a convenient diagnostic test

3) Virulence factors: none significant

4) Epidemiology: transmitted via respiratory droplets

5) Clinical Diseases:

    a) Upper respiratory infections: otitis/sinusitis/bronchitis

    b) **Walking pneumonia**: most commonly affects **teens and young adults**, classic scenario is college dormitory or military barracks, subacute onset over 2–4 weeks of increasingly severe, **nagging, non-productive cough, severity of disease seen on CXR is out of proportion to mild symptoms**, disease is self-limiting in most cases

6) Treatment: macrolide or doxycycline, cell wall inhibitors (e.g., penicillins and cephalosporins) are useless since *Mycoplasma* has no cell wall

7) Resistance: none

8) Prophylaxis: none

f. *Rickettsia spp.*

1) Appearance: tiny rods, do not Gram stain

2) Lab assays: all are obligate intracellular parasites, serologies are the usual diagnostic test, **Weil–Felix test is of historical interest only (detects *Rickettsia* by cross-reaction of anti-rickettsial antibodies to the O-antigen of *Proteus spp.*, and is notoriously unreliable)**

3) Virulence factors: none significant

4) Epidemiology: all are transmitted via bite of arthropods (ticks, fleas, lice)

5) Clinical Diseases:

    a) **Rocky Mountain Spotted Fever**: caused by *R. rickettsii* **transmitted by tick, occurs on east coast of US** (rare in Rocky Mountain states), causes systemic vasculitis with fevers, myalgias, headache, **petechial rash starts on hands and feet and moves in to trunk**, DIC and shock can occur

    b) **Typhus**: scrub typhus transmitted via chiggers, endemic typhus via fleas, epidemic typhus via lice, starts with flu-like symptoms, **petechial rash starts on trunk and moves outward to hands and feet**, vasculitis causes CNS alterations and shock

6) Treatment: doxycycline

7) Resistance: none

8) Prophylaxis: reduction in arthropod populations

TABLE 2.11	Summary of Poorly Stained Bacteria	
ORGANISM	**LAB**	**CHARACTERISTICS**
Actinomyces	Filamentous, weakly gram positive, not acid fast (*Nocardia*)	Look for "sulfur granules," organism causes draining sinus tracts and crosses tissue planes
Intracellular Pathogens		
Chlamydia spp.	Inclusion bodies inside cells	Atypical pneumonia, conjunctivitis, or STD
Coxiella	Serology	Severe headache, pneumonia, hepatitis, acquired by close contact with animal blood/secretions, especially placenta or newborns
Ehrlichia/Anaplasma	Leukocyte inclusion bodies	Leukopenia, thrombocytopenia, transminitis
Mycoplasma	"Fried egg" colony morphology, cold agglutinins positive	Walking pneumonia seen in college-aged people, nagging cough with CXR out of proportion to symptoms
Rickettsia spp.	Weil-Felix test positive	Rocky Mountain spotted fever → petechial rash starting on hands and feet and moving to trunk – Typhus → petechial rash starting on trunk and moving to hands and feet

3. Spirochetal organisms
    a. *Treponema pallidum* (Syphilis)
        1) Appearance: poorly visualized by light microscopy, can visualize by **dark-field microscopy**
        2) Lab assays: cannot be grown in culture, detect by serologies
            a) RPR/VDRL
                i) Detect antibodies to host phospholipids that cross-react to *Treponema* cell surface
                ii) 80% positive in primary disease, 100% in secondary disease, 85% in tertiary disease
                iii) Serology positive acutely but becomes negative with treatment/remission
                iv) **False positives with lupus or other chronic inflammatory diseases**

    b) FTA-ABS
       i)   Antibody directly detects treponemal antigen
       ii) **100% positive in secondary disease, 95% in tertiary disease**
       iii) Positive for life after first exposure, so cannot distinguish between old/treated disease and re-infection
       iv) **Highly specific, minimal false-positive**
3) Virulence factors: none significant
4) Epidemiology: transmitted directly through intact skin or via sexual contact
5) Clinical Diseases:
    a) Primary disease: **chancre = painless ulcer** at site of inoculation, sometimes accompanied by local adenopathy, ulcer heals spontaneously
    b) Secondary disease: almost all untreated patients progress to secondary stage, with **diffuse maculopapular rash that affects palms and soles** (most rashes don't), and development of **moist genital warts called condyloma lata**, bacteremia results in widespread organ seeding including liver/spleen and meninges
    c) Latent syphilis
       i)   One-third of patients spontaneously cure without treatment after secondary disease, 2/3 progress to latent syphilis
       ii) Early latent syphilis is marked by one or more relapses of secondary disease for several years
       iii) Late latent syphilis is asymptomatic persistent disease, develops in 50% of those with early latent syphilis, progresses to tertiary disease
    d) Tertiary syphilis
       i)   **Develops in 1/3 of those initially infected** (2/3 of initially infected get secondary disease, 50% of whom progress to tertiary syphilis)
       ii) **Causes gummas** (erosive ulcerations of bone, skin, or soft tissue), **tabes dorsalis, dementia paralytica, aortitis**
    e) Congenital syphilis: **transmitted transplacentally only after the first trimester, causes snuffles** (bloody nasal discharge), **saber shins, Hutchinson teeth** (notched incisors), saddle nose
6) Treatment: penicillin G or ceftriaxone, **watch out for Jarisch-Herxheimer reaction**, which is rigors and flu-like symptoms after first dose of antibiotics (hypersensitivity reaction to antigens released by bacterial lysis)
7) Resistance: none
8) Prophylaxis: safe sex

b. *Borrelia burgdorferi*
   1) Appearance: visualize by dark-field microscopy or Wright–Giemsa stain
   2) Lab assays: difficult to diagnose, serology and PCR utilized
   3) Virulence factors: none significant
   4) Epidemiology: transmitted via tick bite (*Ixodes scapularis*), endemic to New England area, also more rarely occurs in mountainous areas of California, usually occurs in summer
   5) Clinical Diseases: Lyme disease: starts with erythema chronicum migrans, a spreading bulls-eye rash, within months progresses to myocarditis with heart block, meningitis, and cranial nerve palsies (Bell's is common), over years severe arthritis and dementia/CNS changes occur
   6) Treatment: doxycycline or ceftriaxone
   7) Resistance: none
   8) Prophylaxis: tick repellent, wear long sleeves and pants in wooded areas, vaccine no longer available, consider doxycycline × 1 dose if the tick was attached for >24 h (transmission does not occur in <24 h)
c. *Borrelia recurrentis/hermsii*
   1) Appearance: visualize by **dark-field microscopy** or Wright–Giemsa stain
   2) Lab assays: diagnose by Wright–Giemsa stain of blood
   3) Virulence factors: **antigen phase variation**, due to DNA cassette switching of genes coding for outer membrane antigens,

TABLE 2.12	Summary of Spirochetes	
ORGANISM	**LAB**	**CHARACTERISTICS**
Treponema pallidum	RPR/VDRL for acute disease, FTA is more specific but cannot distinguish acute from old disease	1°dz = chancre; 2°dz = maculopapular rash on palms & soles; 3°dz = gummas, aortitis, CNS dz
Borrelia burgdorferi	Organism may be seen in peripheral blood by Wright–Giemsa stain	Bulls-eye rash, myocarditis, arthritis, CNS/PNS disease
B. recurrentis/hermsii	Organism may be seen in peripheral blood by Wright–Giemsa stain	Recurrent fever alternating with asymptomatic periods
Leptospira	Serology may be helpful	Exposure to animal urine, biphasic illness with hepatitis, renal failure and meningitis

allows the organism to stay one step ahead of the antibody response directed at any one antigen

4) Epidemiology: transmitted via tick or body louse

5) Clinical Diseases: Relapsing fever: causes flu-like illness with lymphadenopathy that lasts for several weeks, then goes away for several weeks, then recurs multiple times (resolution occurs when antibody response catches up to antigen variation, then the organism switches antigen again and the disease relapses)

6) Treatment: doxycycline

7) Resistance: none

8) Prophylaxis: tick repellent, wear long sleeves and pants in wooded areas

d. *Leptospira*

1) Appearance: visualize by **dark-field microscopy**

2) Lab assays: difficult to diagnose, can use serologies

3) Virulence factors: none significant

4) Epidemiology: **transmitted via rat, dog, or cat urine**, organism lives in fresh water, **typical case scenario is people swimming in lake in wilderness area**

5) Clinical Diseases: **Weil's Disease (icterohemorrhagic fever) relapsing fever**: a **biphasic illness** starting with flu-like symptoms followed by resolution for a few days, and then a second phase with diffuse organ involvement, including **hepatitis, acute renal failure, and aseptic meningitis**

6) Treatment: penicillin

7) Resistance: none

8) Prophylaxis: avoid rat, cat, dog, urine—better yet, avoid urine in general!

III. FUNGI

A. Yeast & Dimorphic Fungi

1. Cutaneous & Subcutaneous Pathogens
   a. *Malassezia furfur* AKA *Pityrosporum ovale*
      1) Appearance: KOH prep of skin lesions shows yeast and short hyphae
      2) Lab assays: **fluoresces yellow-green under Woods lamp** (shine the lamp right on the patient's skin, over the macular skin lesions)
      3) Virulence factors: none significant
      4) Epidemiology: ubiquitous, particularly in tropics, transmitted by direct contact or fomites
      5) Clinical Diseases: Tinea versicolor: multiple spherical macules, usually distributed on trunk; **in dark-skinned people the lesions are hypopigmented, in light-skinned people they can be hyperpigmented**
      6) Treatment: topical azole cream
      7) Resistance: none
      8) Prophylaxis: none
   b. *Sporothrix schenckii*
      1) Appearance: KOH prep of skin lesions show **cigar-shaped budding yeast**
      2) Lab assays: in culture at <37°C it grows as a mold, but converts to oval yeast at 37°C
      3) Virulence factors: none significant
      4) Epidemiology: ubiquitous on plants, infection requires antecedent trauma to disrupt the skin barrier, and the **classic scenario (especially on the boards) is infection in a gardener working with rose bushes or anyone suffering a thorn puncture wound**
      5) Clinical Diseases: Sporotrichosis: local nodule forms at the site of inoculation which may ulcerate, and **additional nodules sprout up along the route of lymphatic drainage** on the arm, with localized lymphadenopathy
      6) Treatment: oral potassium iodide (mechanism unclear) or itraconazole
      7) Resistance: none
      8) Prophylaxis: wear protective gloves/clothing while gardening
2. Invasive Pathogens
   a. *Blastomyces dermatitidis*
      1) Appearance: large round yeast with **thick wall and a broad-based bud** (these are key buzzwords on exams!)

TABLE 3.1	Summary of Cutaneous Yeast	
ORGANISM	LAB	CHARACTERISTICS
Malassezia furfur	Lesions fluoresce yellow-green under Woods lamp	Hypopigmented macules in dark-skinned people, hyperpigmented macules in light-skinned people
Sporothrix schenckii	Cigar-shaped yeast on KOH prep	Inoculated by thorn puncturing skin, look for nodules sprouting up in a line along the lymphatics of the arm

2) Lab assays: diagnose by biopsy or smear showing the famous broad-based bud
3) Virulence factors: none significant
4) Epidemiology: almost identical to *Histoplasma* (see below), transmitted via inhalation of spores from soil, is endemic to the Midwestern river valleys and Atlantic states, **key buzz-phrases to look for are travel to the Mississippi, Ohio, or Missouri River valleys, or East Coast/Atlantic states**
5) Clinical Diseases:
   a) Pneumonia: causes a subacute pneumonia similar to histoplasmosis
   b) Disseminated disease: similar to histoplasmosis (see below)
6) Treatment: itraconazole for pneumonia, amphotericin for disseminated disease
7) Resistance: none
8) Prophylaxis: none

b. *Candida spp.*
   1) Appearance: **mucous membrane lesions appear like cottage cheese**, KOH prep of skin lesions show yeast and **pseudohyphae** (germ tubes sprout from yeast but do not form complete hyphae) (see Figure 3.1)
   2) Lab assays: *C. albicans* species can be identified by the germ tube assay, when placed in serum *C. albicans* will form germ tubes within minutes
   3) Virulence factors: avidly adheres to plastic and forms biofilm on plastic so it cannot be eradicated once it is seeded
   4) Epidemiology: normal flora of skin and GI tract, causes thrush in newborns, diabetics, or those with poor T cell-mediated immunity, such as AIDS patients—**intriguingly, it rarely causes invasive disease in patients with T cell defects, but it does cause severe, invasive disease in patients with phagocyte defects (usually neutropenics), and even more interestingly it tends not to cause thrush in these patients**

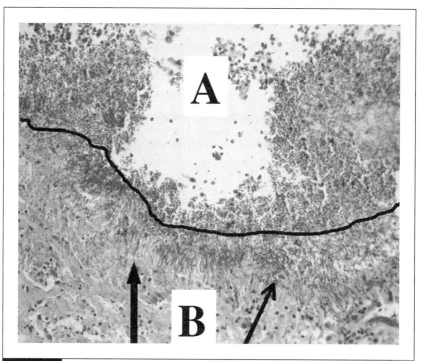

FIGURE 3.1 *Candida* **Invading Tissue**

The slide is artificially divided in half with A) showing the typical necrotic tissue left in the wake of the advancing fungus, and B) showing an advancing line of Candida *hyphae* (thick arrow) *and pseudohyphae* (thin arrow). *Pseudohyphae are intermediate stages between yeast and hyphae, and therefore contain a spherical remnant of the yeast form as well as an elongating protrusion which will develop into the hyphal form. On silver staining, all fungi appear black against a light blue-green background.*

5) Clinical Diseases:
   a) Thrush: mucous membrane infection in young, diabetic, or T cell deficient patients
   b) UTI: seen in nursing home or hospitalized patients, **usually associated with placement of Foley catheter**
   c) Fungemia: **seen in patients with central lines, prolonged ICU stay, neutropenia, patients who have undergone bowel surgery, patients on long-term parenteral nutrition, or patients receiving broad spectrum antibiotics** (wipes out normal flora, allowing *Candida* to proliferate)—mortality in neutropenic patients is 50% even with first-line therapy
   d) Organ seeding: fungemic **patients frequently seed the eye** (always perform funduscopic exam), the liver and spleen

causing microabscesses, the kidney, and can also seed the meninges, iv drug abusers can seed heart valves

6) Treatment:
   a) Thrush: oral fluconazole or topical nystatin swish and swallow
   b) UTI: change or remove the Foley catheter, if necessary treat with oral fluconazole
   c) Fungemia/organ seeding: **remove/change all in-dwelling lines**, in non-neutropenic patients oral fluconazole and iv amphotericin are equivalently efficacious, treat neutropenics with iv amphotericin; caspofungin and voriconazole are now also options for the treatment of candidemia

7) Resistance: **non-albicans species may be resistant to azole drugs**, especially *C. krusei* and *C. glabrata*

8) Prophylaxis: sterile catheter placement, change lines and Foley catheters regularly, avoid broad-spectrum antibiotics if possible

c. *Coccidioides immitis*
   1) Appearance: **giant spherules with thick walls, filled with dozens of smaller endospores, particularly visible on silver stain** (see Figure 3.2)

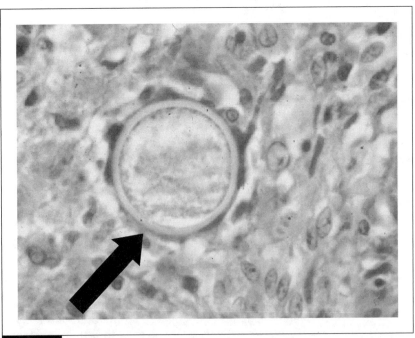

FIGURE 3.2 A Giant *Coccidioides* Spherule Seen in Tissue

The spherule contains dozens of yeast forms within its tough walls.

2) Lab assays: grows as mold in soil but spherule in tissue, diagnose by biopsy or serology, culturing poses hazards to lab personnel
3) Virulence factors: none significant
4) Epidemiology: transmitted via inhalation of spores which grow in soil in **southwestern U.S.** (central and southern California, especially desert areas, New Mexico, Arizona, Texas), **look for several key buzz-phrases in exam questions: travel to southwestern U.S. desert, archaeological expedition** (due to close contact with soil), **time proximity to earthquake** (disruption of soil by shaking often causes outbreaks)
5) Clinical Diseases:
   a) Pneumonia: San Joaquin Valley fever (named for a valley in Central California): usually occurs in people traveling through the southwestern U.S. (not natives), presents with **TB-like constitutional symptoms**, fevers, weight loss, chronic cough, and also can present with **erythema nodosum** (good prognostic sign**), CXR shows infiltrate with hilar adenopathy**
   b) Disseminated disease: **increased likelihood in African-Americans and Filipinos** (for unclear reasons, but known not to be linked to MHC), as well as in immunocompromised patients, causes disseminated skin lesions, as well as hepatosplenic granulomas, and can disseminate to meninges causing severe meningitis, look for hypercalcemia (a sign of disseminated granulomatous disease)
6) Treatment: fluconazole
7) Resistance: none
8) Prophylaxis: avoid southwestern desert areas
d. *Cryptococcus neoformans*
   1) Appearance: oval budding yeast with large capsule (see Figure 3.3)
   2) Lab assays: **India Ink preparation (especially of CSF) reveals small spherical organism surrounded by giant white "halo"** which is the polysaccharide capsule, can also send CSF and serum for CRAG (cryptococcal antigen)
   3) Virulence factors: polysaccharide capsule inhibits phagocytosis
   4) Epidemiology: transmitted via aerosolization of **pigeon droppings** (or other birds)
   5) Clinical Diseases: Meningitis: **usually in AIDS patients but non-AIDS patients do develop the disease if organism burden is high enough** (consider the diagnosis in a case scenario involving a pigeon farmer!), disease disseminates in AIDS patients, causing skin lesions and organ seeding
   6) Treatment: amphotericin plus flucytosine intravenously, followed by oral fluconazole suppression
   7) Resistance: none

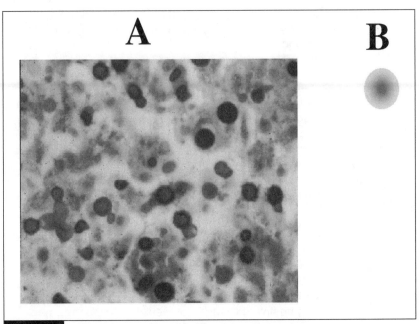

FIGURE 3.3 *Cryptococcus* **Yeast in Tissues**

A) Cryptococcus *yeast in tissues. B) In CSF, India ink stain reveals yeast surrounded by a think, clear, polysaccharide capsule. The India ink does not stain the polysaccharide, leaving the appearance of a "halo" around the yeast.*

8) Prophylaxis: no primary prophylaxis (except to avoid pigeon guano!), but all patients who develop the disease should receive chronic fluconazole for secondary prophylaxis

e. *Histoplasma capsulatum*
   1) Appearance: biopsy shows oval yeast, sometimes found within macrophages (see Figure 3.4)
   2) Lab assays: **urine *Histoplasma* antigen is highly reliable**, organism grows as mold in soil but spherule in tissue
   3) Virulence factors: none significant
   4) Epidemiology: transmitted via inhalation of spores which are carried at **high burdens in bat guano and bird droppings**, is endemic to the Midwestern river valleys, **key buzz-phrases to look for are exposure to bats, spelunking expedition (people who climb in caves and get exposed to bats), travel to the Mississippi, Ohio, or Missouri River Valleys, or the patient recently cleaned his/her chicken coops**
   5) Clinical Diseases:
      a) Pneumonia: causes a subacute pneumonia similar to *Coccidioides* and TB, **CXR shows infiltrates and hilar adenopathy**

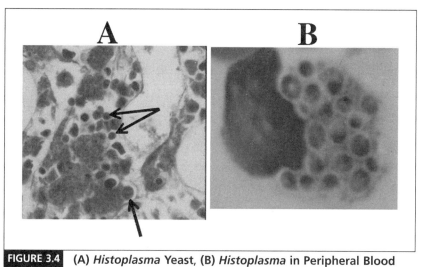

FIGURE 3.4 (A) *Histoplasma* Yeast, (B) *Histoplasma* in Peripheral Blood

A) Appearance of Histoplasma *yeast (arrows) in a section of lung. B) Appearance of a clump of* Histoplasma *in peripheral blood.*

    b) Disseminated disease: occurs in immunocompromised, like *Cocci* it causes disseminated skin lesions, as well as hepatosplenic granulomas; it can disseminate to any organ

6) Treatment: itraconazole for pneumonia, amphotericin for disseminated disease

7) Resistance: none

8) Prophylaxis: avoid bat guano, be careful when cleaning chicken coops, be wary while on those frequent spelunking expeditions

f. *Pneumocystis jiroveci* (formerly known as *P. carinii*, however still okay to refer to pneumonia as PCP, standing for P̲neumo̲c̲ystis p̲neumonia; an editorial has been published recommending this, since the term PCP is so ingrained in clinical practice)

1) Appearance: clumps of cysts best seen on silver staining (see Figure 3.5)

2) Lab assays: silver stain and culture of bronchoscopic washings are necessary for the diagnosis

3) Virulence factors: none significant

4) Epidemiology: ubiquitous fungus, which almost always **causes disease in AIDS patients or patients on chronic steroids**

5) Clinical Diseases: Pneumonia (PCP): typically a subacute presentation followed by a sudden decompensation in function, **with severe hypoxia and dyspnea out of proportion to unimpressive lung exam, CXR shows "ground glass" haziness in bilateral lower lobes, pleural effusions are distinctly rare**

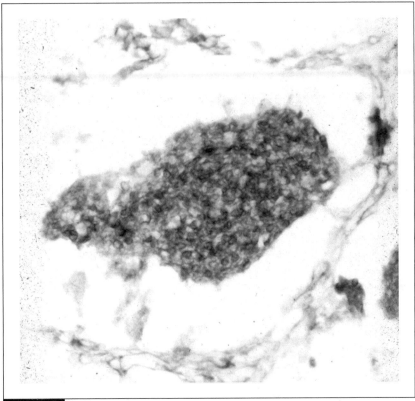

FIGURE 3.5 *Pneumocystis*

Silver stain revealing a large clump of Pneumocystis *within an alveola.*

and their presence should make one reconsider the diagnosis, patients typically have markedly elevated **LDH** which comes down with treatment
6) Treatment: intravenous trimethoprim-sulfamethoxazole plus prednisone taper
7) Resistance: unusual
8) Prophylaxis: **all AIDS patients with CD4 counts <200 should be on trimethoprim-sulfamethoxazole prophylaxis**

B. Molds

1. Cutaneous Pathogens
   a. Dermatophytes (*Microsporum, Trichophyton, Epidermophyton*)
      1) Appearance: KOH prep of skin lesions show hyphae
      2) Lab assays: none significant

TABLE 3.2	Summary of Invasive Yeast	
	APPEARANCE	**EPIDEMIOLOGY**
Candida	Pseudohyphae	Normal flora, risk factors for fungemia: (1) catheters, (2) long ICU stay, (3) GI surgery, (4) broad spectrum antibiotics, (5) neutropenia, (6) parenteral nutrition
Cryptococcus	Giant halo in India ink	Aerosolized pigeon droppings, usually in AIDS
Coccidioides	Giant spherules filled with endospores	Inhaled spores from soil in SW U.S. states, ↑ risk dissemination in African American and Filipinos
Histoplasma	Oval yeast within macrophages	Inhalation of spores in bat or bird guano, endemic to Midwestern river valleys, spelunking is high risk
Blastomyces	Thick-walled yeast with broad-based bud	Inhalation of spores from soil, endemic to Midwestern river valleys and Atlantic states
Pneumocystis	Silver-stained cysts	Ubiquitous, causes disease in AIDS or other T cell deficiency (e.g., steroid treatment)

        3) Virulence factors: none significant

        4) Epidemiology: ubiquitous, spread by direct contact or fomites

        5) Clinical Diseases: cause the common conditions of athlete's foot (tinea pedis), jock-itch (tinea cruris), and ringworm

        6) Treatment: topical azole cream

        7) Resistance: none

        8) Prophylaxis: good hygiene

  2. Invasive Pathogens

    a. *Aspergillus fumigatus*

      1) Appearance: **septate hyphae with branching at 45° angles** (see Figure 3.6)

      2) Lab assays: IgE titers for *Aspergillus* are high in allergic bronchopulmonary Aspergillosis; invasive disease is diagnosed by a combination of clinical risk factors, radiology (i.e., the "halo sign" on CT scan, which is a nodule, often cavitating, surrounded by hypodense lung), and tissue biopsy

      3) Virulence factors: none significant

      4) Epidemiology: ubiquitous organism, transmission is airborne via soil or fresh vegetation

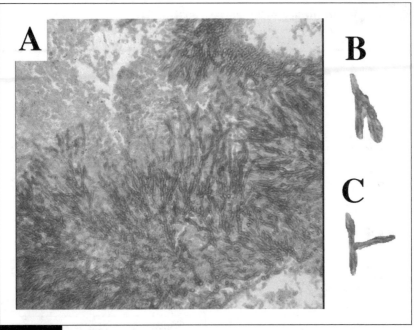

FIGURE 3.6 *Aspergillus* vs. *Mucor*

A) Aspergillus *hyphae invading lung tissue.* Aspergillus *causes extensive tissue necrosis, visible in the upper left corner of the image. B) A close-up image of an individual* Aspergillus *hyphus, revealing the characteristic 45° angle at which the hyphae branch. C) For comparison, a 90° angle of branching typical of the mold,* Mucor.

5) Clinical Diseases:
   a) **Fungus ball:** the organism **colonizes cavities formed by prior necrotizing disease, commonly from old tuberculosis,** and causes hemoptysis, rarely becomes invasive
   b) Invasive Pulmonary Aspergillosis: **seen in neutropenic patients or those on chronic steroids,** casing hemoptysis, dyspnea, and even pneumothorax, as disease progresses hypoxia can become severe
   c) Allergic Bronchopulmonary Aspergillosis: **a hypersensitivity reaction to fungus** in the large airways, acts very similar to asthma, high titers of IgE specific for the organism are helpful in diagnosis
   d) Disseminated disease: **usually in neutropenics,** or patients on chronic steroids, can seed any organ, highly lethal
6) Treatment:
   a) Fungus ball: none vs. itraconazole/voriconazole suppression vs. resection for refractory hemoptysis

   b) Invasive Pulmonary Aspergillosis: voriconazole is now
      considered 1st line, with amphotericin B second line, and
      caspofungin also useful
   c) Allergic Bronchopulmonary Aspergillosis: itraconazole
   d) Disseminated disease: voriconazole ± amphotericin B ±
      caspofungin—disseminated disease has a mortality of
      >50% even with therapy
7) Resistance: not intrinsically resistant to amphotericin B
   in vitro, but difficult to treat *in vivo*
8) Prophylaxis: neutropenic precautions = strict hand-washing,
   no fresh fruits or vegetables, no intramuscular injections, etc.
b. Mucormycosis (*Mucor* and *Rhizopus*)
   1) Appearance: **nonseptate hyphae with branching at 90° angles**
      (see Figure 3.6C)
   2) Lab assays: diagnosis made by tissue biopsy
   3) Virulence factors: none significant
   4) Epidemiology: ubiquitous on decaying vegetation, can be
      transmitted via inhalation or direct skin contact
   5) Clinical Diseases:
      a) **Rhinocerebral mucormycosis is almost exclusively seen in
         diabetic patients in ketoacidosis** (the acidity is the key to
         susceptibility, not just high glucose), a deadly, invasive
         disease usually starting in the sinuses which erodes through
         the skull, into the eyes and brain, typically presents
         (especially on the boards) with a bad headache or acute
         vision change in a diabetic in ketoacidosis—**always think
         of *Mucor* in a diabetic with a headache or vision change**
      b) Pulmonary or disseminated disease, typically seen in neutro-
         penic patients or those on high dose immunosuppression
   6) Treatment: surgical resection and amphotericin B, the
      amphotericin alone only halts the spread to further tissue,
      but does nothing for already infected tissue
   7) Resistance: variable susceptibility to amphotericin B, very
      difficult to treat *in vivo*
   8) Prophylaxis: none

TABLE 3.3	**Summary of Invasive Molds**	
	APPEARANCE	**EPIDEMIOLOGY**
Aspergillus	Septate hyphae, 45° branches	Neutropenics and chronic steroid
Mucormycosis	Non-septate hyphae, 90° branches	Diabetic ketoacidosis and neutropenics

TABLE 3.4	**Overall Summary of Fungi**	
	KEY WORD/PHRASES	**TREATMENT**
Cutaneous Yeast		
Malassezia	• Tinea versicolor • Fluoresces under Woods lamp	Topical azole cream
Sporothrix	• Inoculated via thorn puncture of skin • Spreads up lymphatics of arm	Potassium iodide or itraconazole
Invasive Yeast		
Blastomyces	• Microscope → "thick wall, broad-based bud" • Indigenous to Midwestern river valleys and Atlantic states • Very similar to *Histoplasma*	Itraconazole (not fluconazole), amphotericin for disseminated disease
Candida	• Cottage cheese appearance • Risk for mucosal dz = T cell defects (AIDS) • Risks for invasive dz = neutropenia, ICU, multiple catheters, broad-spectrum antibiotics, GI surgery	Fluconazole for non-neutropenics, amphotericin B for neutropenics
Coccidioides	• Indigenous to Southwestern U.S. deserts • Exposure to soil (e.g., archaeological expedition or yard work) and time proximity to earthquakes • Mimics TB clinically • Hilar adenopathy and erythema nodosum • Filipinos and African Americans much higher risk of developing disseminated dz	Fluconazole or amphotericin (for severe disease)

TABLE 3.4	Continued	
	KEY WORD/PHRASES	**TREATMENT**
Cryptococcus	• Meningitis in AIDS patients • India ink test positive in CSF • Pigeon droppings loaded with *Cryptococcus*	Amphotericin, then fluconazole for life
Histoplasma	• Indigenous to Midwestern river valleys • Bat and bird guano contain the organism • Exposure to caves (e.g., spelunking) or cleaning of chicken coops • Like *Cocci*, mimics TB	Itraconazole (not fluconazole), amphotericin for disseminated disease
Pneumocystis	• Silver stain of bronchoscopy makes dx • Almost always in AIDS pts • Insidious dyspnea with abrupt decline in course • CXR shows "ground glass" haziness • Markedly elevated LDH	Bactrim plus prednisone
	Cutaneous Molds	
Microsporum, Trichophyton, Epidermophyton	• Athlete's foot • Jock itch • Ringworm	Topical azole cream
	Invasive Molds	
Aspergillus	• Septate hyphae with 45° branches • Fungus ball on CXR • Neutropenia almost always present	Voriconazole 1st line
Mucormycosis	• Non-septate hyphae with 90° branches • Ketoacidosis most common risk • Also seen in neutropenics • Starts with subtle headache or visual loss	Surgery plus amphotericin B

IV. PARASITES

A. Protozoa

1. GI/GU
   a. *Cryptosporidium*
      1) Appearance: cysts are small, **stain pink in stool specimens**
      2) Lab assays: stool O&P
      3) Virulence factors: none significant
      4) Epidemiology: ubiquitous but **typically causes disease in AIDS patients**
      5) Clinical Diseases: watery diarrhea, causes severe malabsorption in AIDS patients
      6) Treatment: supportive and immune reconstitution—nitazoxanide may have a role
      7) Resistance: none
      8) Prophylaxis: boil or filter water, chlorination does not work
   b. *Entamoeba histolytica*
      1) Appearance: two phases of life-cycle: cyst has four nuclei, trophozoite has one nucleus and is not flagellated and often contains ingested red blood cells (see Figure 4.1)
      2) Lab assays: stool O&P should reveal cyst or trophozoite, anti-amoeba antibody titers are diagnostically useful
      3) Virulence factors: none significant
      4) Epidemiology: fecal-oral transmission
      5) Clinical Diseases: amoebic dysentery and amoebic liver abscess
      6) Treatment: metronidazole followed by iodoquinol or paromomycin—the latter are necessary to kill encysted organisms in the bowel lumen that are not killed by metronidazole
      7) Resistance: none
      8) Prophylaxis: boil or filter water, chlorination has no effect, careful hand-washing and separation of human wastes from crop fields (don't fertilize crops with human feces)
   c. *Giardia lamblia*
      1) Appearance: two phases of life cycle: cyst has four nuclei and has a thicker wall than *Entamoeba*, **trophozoite is oval with two nuclei and has four pairs of flagella** (see Figure 4.2)
      2) Lab assays: stool O&P, string test = patient swallows a string down into the duodenum while the physician holds onto the far end and then pulls the string back up out of the mouth, revealing the trophozoites stuck onto the string
      3) Virulence factors: none significant
      4) Epidemiology: fecal-oral transmission, often via streams in the wilderness as many animals carry *Giardia* as well, **classic**

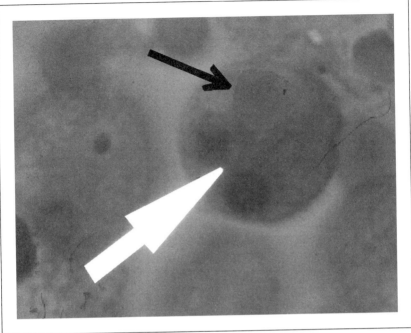

FIGURE 4.1 Classic *Entamoeba* Cyst

Classic Entamoeba *cyst (light arrow) with an ingested red blood cell (dark arrow).*

Boards scenario is a hiker who drinks from a stream and gets diarrhea, disease is common in patients with IgA deficiency

5) Clinical Diseases: chronic diarrhea, no tissue invasive disease

6) Treatment: metronidazole

7) Resistance: none

8) Prophylaxis: boiling or filtering water, chlorination doesn't work

d. *Trichomonas*

1) Appearance: there is no cyst stage, **pear-shaped trophozoite, with four flagella, highly motile on wet mount**

2) Lab assays: wet mount

3) Virulence factors: none significant

4) Epidemiology: sexually transmitted, resides in the vagina or, rarely in male GU tract, can be spread by asymptomatic carriers

5) Clinical Diseases: vaginitis with **green, frothy discharge,** can cause urethritis in men, **watch out for Boards questions where both the male and female sex partners have GU symptoms, or questions in which the female is diagnosed with** *Trichomonas* **and treated appropriately but comes back**

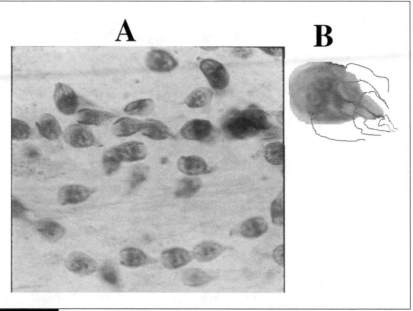

FIGURE 4.2 *Giardia* **Trophozoites**

A) Typical appearance of Giardia *trophozoites from an intestinal biopsy. B) Close-up of an individual trophozoite, revealing the presence of two nuclei and four pairs of flagella.*

   shortly with a new infection—both sex partners must be treated simultaneously to eradicate the disease

  6) Treatment: metronidazole, treat both sex partners

  7) Resistance: none

  8) Prophylaxis: condoms

 2. Invasive protozoa

  a. *Babesia*

   1) Appearance: intracellular ring forms within red cells similar to malaria

   2) Lab assays: blood smear, serology

   3) Virulence factors: none significant

   4) Epidemiology: transmitted via tick bite, **typically occurs in the New England area, specifically along the coast**

   5) Clinical Diseases: high fevers, shaking chills, myalgias, abdominal pain, nausea/vomiting, followed by **severe hemolytic anemia particularly dangerous in splenectomized patients**

   6) Treatment: clindamycin plus quinine

   7) Resistance: none

   8) Prophylaxis: avoid tick bites

ORGANISM	APPEARANCE	DISEASE	TREATMENT
TABLE 4.1	**Summary of GI/GU Protozoa**		
Cryptosporidium	Cyst stain pink in stool, nuclei not visible	Watery diarrhea, typically in AIDS	Immune reconstitution
Entamoeba	Thin-walled cyst with 4 nuclei, **trophozoite ingests red blood cells and is not flagellated**	Bloody diarrhea, invasive hepatic abscess	Metronidazole and iodoquinol
Giardia	Thick-walled cyst with 4 nuclei, **trophozoite is oval and has 4 pairs of flagella**	Non-bloody diarrhea, often in hikers	Metronidazole
Trichomonas	No cyst, **trophozoite is oval with 4 single flagella**	Vaginitis	Metronidazole (treat both sex partners)

b. *Leishmania spp.*
   1) Appearance: amastigotes are small intracellular organisms seen within macrophages
   2) Lab assays: blood smear or tissue biopsy reveal organisms within macrophages, serologies often positive
   3) Virulence factors: none significant
   4) Epidemiology: transmitted via sandfly bite, visceral disease seen in Asia and Africa, cutaneous disease seen in Central and South America as well as Asia and Africa, mucocutaneous disease seen only in Central and South America
   5) Clinical Diseases:
      a) **Kala azar = visceral leishmaniasis: caused by *L. donovani*,** organism is concentrated in the reticuloendothelial system (liver, spleen, lymph nodes, bone marrow), causing **massive hepatosplenomegaly, pancytopenia,** hemorrhage, and susceptibility to secondary infections, patients also get hyperpigmented skin
      b) **Cutaneous leishmaniasis: caused by *L. tropica*** (Old World disease in Asia and Africa) and ***L. mexicana*** (New World disease in Central/South America), disease starts with **erythematous papule at site of sandfly bite,** can either heal spontaneously or progress to large, granulomatous ulcerations which often is secondarily infected by bacteria
      c) **Mucocutaneous leishmaniasis: caused by *L. braziliensis*, also starts as papule at site of sandfly bite,** but can

disseminate to multiple mucosal spots, creating granulomatous erosions of nose and mouth
6) Treatment: sodium stibogluconate, ketoconazole, liposomal
amphotericin B, miltefosine
7) Resistance: unusual
8) Prophylaxis: long-sleeve shirts, long pants, insect repellents,
pesticides to kill sandflies
c. *Plasmodium* (malaria): *falciparum, vivax, ovale, malariae*
1) Appearance: schizonts appear like **"signet rings"** in red blood
cells, while the gametocyte of *P. falciparum* appears like a
large crescent attached to a thin ring (see Figure 4.3)
2) Lab assays: thin and thick smear of whole blood to detect
trophozoites
3) Virulence factors: none significant
4) Epidemiology: **transmitted by bite of *Anopheles* mosquito,
infects several hundred million people worldwide**, particularly affects Africa and all Mediterranean countries, **causes
about 1 million deaths per year**, life cycle is complicated:

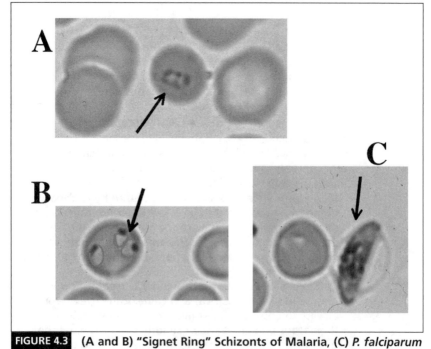

FIGURE 4.3   **(A and B) "Signet Ring" Schizonts of Malaria, (C)** *P. falciparum*

*A) and B) show typical "signet ring" schizonts of malaria in red blood cells.
C) shows the classic "crescent" shaped gametocyte of* P. falciparum *found in
peripheral blood.*

sporozoites inoculated into blood from mosquito bite, seed the liver and transform into merozoites, leave the liver and infect red blood cells, transform into trophozoite which multiplies and then transforms back into merozoites and bursts the red cell, infects new red cells and then the cycle repeats—note that *P. ovale* and *P. vivax* can lie dormant in the liver, allowing long-term relapse

5) Clinical Diseases:
   a) General characteristics: all four species cause a cluster of symptoms including **paroxysmal fevers and shaking rigors, myalgias, diaphoresis, severe headache, arthralgias, and signs such as splenomegaly and hepatomegaly, red cell lysis causes anemia, initially the fever is continuous, but after several days the red cell bursts become synchronized in *P. vivax, ovale*, and *malariae* infections, note that *falciparum* may never become synchronized**
   b) **Tertian fever:** synchronous red cell bursts in *P. vivax* and *ovale* cause tertian fevers (q48 hrs = tertian because it occurs on the 3rd day, it is not q3 days), **relapse is common in tertian fever because *vivax* and *ovale* have a latent phase in the liver**
   c) **Quartan fever:** synchronous red cell bursts in *P. malariae* causes quartan fevers (**q72 hrs** because it occurs on the 4th day, it is not q4 days)
   d) *P. falciparum* **causes the most severe malaria, can cause continuous or irregular fevers without patterns, the organism burden in *P. falciparum* infections is much higher, and the red cells become sticky and can clog capillaries and cause DIC, leading to strokes and renal failure, CNS disease in a malaria patient is almost always due to *P. falciparum*, and carries a very high mortality**

6) Treatment:
   a) Tertian fever: **if *P. vivax* or *ovale* proven or suspected, treat with chloroquine (for merozoites in blood) plus primaquine (for latent organisms in liver)**—beware pts with G6PDH deficiency, in whom quinine-derivatives cause dangerous hemolytic anemia
   b) *P. falciparum* and Quartan fever: if *P. falciparum* or *malariae* proven or suspected, treat with chloroquine alone (primaquine not needed since there is no latent liver phase)—beware pts with G6PDH deficiency

7) Resistance: an increasingly severe problem, resistance endemic in South America, Africa, SE Asia, and parts of Middle East with few proven alternatives to quinine-derivatives, quinine plus doxycycline may cover some resistant organisms, other regimens are so unusual they are not likely testable on the USMLE

TABLE 4.2	Summary of *Plasmodium spp.*			
ORGANISM	**FEVER TIMING**	**CNS Dz**	**LATENT?**	**TREATMENT***
Falciparum	Irregular or q48 hr	Yes	No	CQ
Vivaxlovale	q48 hr	No	Yes	CQ + PQ
Malariae	q72 hr	No	No	CQ

*Assumes not resistant.
CQ, chloroquine; PQ, primaquine.

8) Prophylaxis:
   a) Mosquito netting and DEET insect repellent are keys to avoid inoculation—it is much more effective to prevent bites than to treat infection due to increasing drug resistance
   b) Chemoprophylaxis depends on if travel is to area with resistant organism
      i) Non-resistant area (Central America north of the Panama Canal, some parts of the Middle East and some parts of the Caribbean): chloroquine for several weeks before the trip, during the trip, and for several weeks after the trip
      ii) Resistant area: mefloquine, atovaquone-proguanil, or doxycycline before, during the trip, and after the trip
d. *Toxoplasma gondii*
   1) Appearance: biopsy of infected tissue reveals crescent-shaped organisms
   2) Lab assays: IgM serologies to detect acute infection
   3) Virulence factors: none significant
   4) Epidemiology: **transmitted via the feces of kittens (older cats less likely),** or via ingestion of poorly cooked meat containing cysts, can also be transmitted vertically if the mother is newly infected during pregnancy
   5) Clinical Diseases:
      a) Immunocompetent people either get asymptomatically exposed or develop **mild heterophile negative mononucleosis**
      b) AIDS patients: **clinical disease primarily seen in HIV patients,** immunosuppression allows reactivation of the organism, classically causing severe **encephalitis with multiple ring-enhancing lesions in the brain**
      c) Congenital: causes multi-organ disease and can lead to spontaneous abortion or severe congenital retardation
   6) Treatment: pyrimethamine plus sulfadiazine plus folinic acid (folinic acid is used to prevent folate deficiency caused by the drugs—**note that folate cannot be used because folate is**

upstream of the drug-induced block in the biosynthetic pathway, folinic acid is used because it is downstream of the block)

7) Resistance: none, but alternative therapies are required in sulfa-allergic patients

8) Prophylaxis: AIDS patients and pregnant women should avoid kittens and should not clean kitty litter, cook meats thoroughly, **AIDS patients with CD4 count <200 per μL should be on trimethoprim-sulfamethoxazole prophylaxis**

e. *Trypanosoma*

1) Appearance: large, crescentic trypomastigotes seen in blood, smaller, circular amastigotes seen in tissues

2) Lab assays: biopsy and serologies

3) Virulence factors: **antigenic shift**—the organism can shift its surface antigens as antibody responses develop, keeping it one step ahead of the immune response

4) Epidemiology: *T. cruzi* **transmitted via reduviid bug**, endemic to Central and South America, which bites the patient and then passes organism through the broken skin by defecating in the bite wound, *T. gambiense* and *T. rhodesiense* **transmitted by the tsetse fly, endemic to Africa**

5) Clinical Diseases:

a) Chagas disease: caused by *T. cruzi*, **reduviid bug often bites the face near the eyes, so look for Romana's sign, a swollen/puffy cheek near the eye**, acutely the organism causes lymphoreticular disease with fever, lymphadenopathy, and hepatosplenomegaly, chronic persistence of the organism leads to amastigote invasion of the heart and colon, **causing heart block and myocarditis/dilated cardiomyopathy as well as megacolon, and achalasia**

b) African Sleeping Sickness: caused by *T. gambiense* and *T. rhodesiense*, presents with an ulcer at the site of the fly bite, **can lead to either an acute, severe encephalitis with rapid decline in CNS function leading to coma, or a chronic course over several years**

6) Treatment:

a) Chagas disease: if caught during acute infection, nifurtimox effective, there is no antimicrobial therapy for chronic disease; however, **pacemakers are crucial if heart block develops**

b) African Sleeping Sickness: **suramin or melarsoprol may be effective prior to onset of CNS disease** but they don't cross the blood brain barrier well, so useless once CNS disease sets in

7) Resistance: unusual

8) Prophylaxis: insect netting, insect repellent

TABLE 4.3	**Summary of Invasive Protozoa**		
	TRANSMISSION	**EPIDEMIOLOGY**	**TISSUE TROPISM**
Babesia	Tick bite	• Coastal New England	Red blood cells
Leishmania	Sandfly bite	• Mucocutaneous dz in Central/South America	Macrophages
		• Cutaneous dz in Central/South America & Asia/Africa	
		• Visceral dz in Asia/Africa	
Plasmodium	*Anopheles* mosquito	Africa, Middle East, Caribbean, Central/ South America, SE Asia	RBCs (liver for *P. vivax/ovale*)
Toxoplasma	Cat feces or cysts in undercooked meat	Ubiquitous	Brain
Trypanosoma	• Reduviid bug (*cruzi*)	• Central/South America (*cruzi*)	Heart (*cruzi*), CNS (other *spp*)
	• Tsetse fly (other *spp*)	• Africa (other *spp*)	

B. Metazoa (Multicellular Animals)

1. Tapeworms (cestodes)
   a. *Diphyllobothrium latum*
      1) Appearance: **longest tapeworm,** up to 30 feet
      2) Lab assays: stool O&P
      3) Virulence factors: none significant
      4) Epidemiology: **acquired by consuming raw, freshwater fish**
      5) Clinical Diseases: weight loss, diarrhea, **vitamin B12 deficiency**
      6) Treatment: praziquantel/niclosamide
      7) Resistance: none
      8) Prophylaxis: cook fish
   b. *Echinococcus*
      1) Appearance: small tapeworm
      2) Lab assays: stool O&P
      3) Virulence factors: none significant
      4) Epidemiology: fecal oral transmission from **dog feces, with sheep an important intermediate host—thus shepherds are commonly patients**
      5) Clinical Diseases: hydatid cysts in any organ of the body, if cysts rupture can cause fatal anaphylaxis

6) Treatment: careful surgical excystation with or without albendazole
7) Resistance: none
8) Prophylaxis: good hygiene

c. *Hymenolepis nana*
   1) Appearance: small tapeworm (up to 5 cm long)
   2) Lab assays: stool O&P
   3) Virulence factors: none significant
   4) Epidemiology: fecal oral transmission, with humans as major host
   5) Clinical Diseases: typically asymptomatic
   6) Treatment: praziquantel/niclosamide
   7) Resistance: none
   8) Prophylaxis: good hygiene

d. *Taenia saginata* (beef tapeworm)
   1) Appearance: tapeworm can be several meters long
   2) Lab assays: stool O&P
   3) Virulence factors: none significant
   4) Epidemiology: **ingestion of undercooked beef**, transmitted to cattle via fecal-oral route
   5) Clinical Diseases: typically asymptomatic, although some patients might suffer discomfort (and embarrassment!) due to the **occasional protrusion of the tapeworm tail from the anus**
   6) Treatment: praziquantel/niclosamide
   7) Resistance: none
   8) Prophylaxis: good hygiene

e. *Taenia solium* (pork tapeworm)
   1) Appearance: tapeworm can be several meters long
   2) Lab assays: stool O&P
   3) Virulence factors: none significant
   4) Epidemiology: **can be transmitted either by ingestion of larva in undercooked pork causing tapeworm infection of gut, or by ingestion of eggs in food due to fecal contamination**, eggs mature into larva in gut and burrow into tissues, causing cysticercosis
   5) Clinical Diseases:
      a) Tapeworm infection: like *T. saginata*, often asymptomatic
      b) Cysticercosis: space-occupying lesions occur in tissues, often in brain, and death of the larva induces inflammatory response which can cause seizures and chemical meningitis— **new onset seizures in an immigrant from Latin America is neurocysticercosis until proven otherwise**
   6) Treatment: seizure medications, steroids for edema, with or without albendazole or praziquantel

TABLE 4.4	Summary of Tapeworms (cestodes)	
	TRANSMISSION	**CLINICAL Dz**
Diphyllobothrium	Raw fish	Weight loss, diarrhea, B12 deficiency
Echinococcus	Dog feces or ingestion of infected sheep meat	Causes anaphylaxis when cysts rupture often after trauma/traffic accident
Hymenolepis	Human feces	Asymptomatic
Taenia saginata	Undercooked beef	Typically asymptomatic, worm may protrude from anus
Taenia solium	Undercooked pork or human feces	Asymptomatic tapeworm infection, or ingestion of eggs in feces causes cysticercosis, which presents with seizures and chemical meningitis from ruptured cysts in the brain

      7) Resistance: none

      8) Prophylaxis: good hygiene

2. Flukes (trematodes)

   a. *Clonorchis sinensis* (**Asian liver fluke**)

      1) Appearance: not remarkable

      2) Lab assays: stool O&P

      3) Virulence factors: none significant

      4) Epidemiology: **transmitted by ingestion of raw freshwater fish, endemic to Asia**

      5) Clinical Diseases: may be asymptomatic, however, the flukes lodge in the liver and can cause **hepatitis and biliary obstruction** ultimately leading to cirrhosis or hepatocellular carcinoma

      6) Treatment: praziquantel/albendazole

      7) Resistance: none

      8) Prophylaxis: cook fish

   b. *Paragonimus westermani* (**Asian lung fluke**)

      1) Appearance: not remarkable

      2) Lab assays: stool O&P

      3) Virulence factors: none significant

      4) Epidemiology: transmitted by **ingestion of raw crab meat, endemic to Asia**, organism penetrates intestinal wall, migrates through the diaphragm to the lung and can thus be transmitted either by feces or sputum

5) Clinical Diseases: chronic cough, hemoptysis and dyspnea
6) Treatment: praziquantel
7) Resistance: none
8) Prophylaxis: cook crab meat

c. *Schistosoma japonicum, mansoni,* and *haematobium*
  1) Appearance: ova are ovoid with sharp protuberance called a spine at one end, *S. haematobium* ova have a big spine at the very terminus of the egg, *S. mansoni* ovum have big spine off to the side (about 2 o'clock if the terminus is 12 noon), while *S. japonicum* have a less prominent spine (see Figure 4.4)
  2) Lab assays: stool O&P
  3) Virulence factors: none significant
  4) Epidemiology:
     a) Infection occurs by direct **penetration of human skin by free-swimming larva, life-cycle requires freshwater environment with snails** (which are intermediate hosts)
     b) *S. mansoni* occurs in tropical areas around the world, including Africa, the Middle East, and South America, but **does not occur in Asia**
     c) *S. japonicum* **occurs in Asia**
     d) *S. haematobium* occurs in Africa and the Middle East

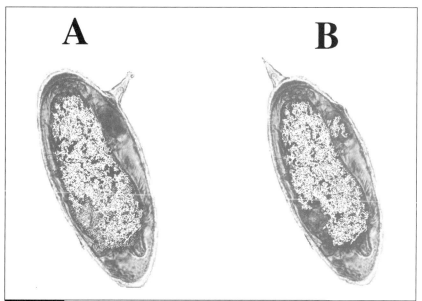

FIGURE 4.4   **(A)** *Schistosoma mansoni*, **(B)** *Schistosoma haematobium*

A) The classic appearance of Schistosoma mansoni, *with a terminal spine at approximately 2 o'clock. B) In contrast, the spine of* Schistosoma haematobium *is at the very terminus (12 o'clock).*

TABLE 4.5 Summary of Flukes (trematodes)			
	TRANSMISSION	**LOCATION**	**CLINICAL Dz**
Clonorchis	Raw freshwater fish	Asia	Hepatitis, biliary obstruction
Paragonimus	Raw crab meat	Asia	Chronic cough, hemoptysis
Schistosoma haematobium	Skin penetration by freshwater larvae	Africa, Middle East	Hematuria, transitional bladder CA
Schistosoma japonicum	Skin penetration by freshwater larvae	Asia	Granulomatous hepatitis, cirrhosis, portal hypertension
Schistosoma mansoni	Skin penetration by freshwater larvae	Africa, Middle East, South America	Granulomatous hepatitis, cirrhosis, portal hypertension

    5) Clinical Diseases:
       a) *S. japonicum* & *mansoni*: acute infection **causes pruritis and erythematous eruption at the site of skin penetration,** after several weeks fevers and lymphadenopathy begin, tissue penetration causes **marked eosinophilia, adult schistosomes reside in the liver venules and their eggs cause granulomatous reaction in the liver, leading to portal hypertension and hepatosplenomegaly, can induce cirrhosis** leading to all the usual sequelae
       b) *S. hematobium*: **adult worms reside in the bladder venous plexus,** and their eggs cause granulomas and fibrosis in the bladder, leading to **hematuria, can also induce transitional cell carcinoma of the bladder**
    6) Treatment: praziquantel
    7) Resistance: starting to be seen for *S. mansoni*
    8) Prophylaxis: avoid swimming in waters with host snails

  3. Intestinal Roundworms (nematodes)
    a. *Ascaris lumbricoides*
      1) Appearance: large roundworms, can be a foot long, and can form mass-like conglomerations in the intestines (see Figure 4.5)
      2) Lab assays: stool O&P
      3) Virulence factors: none significant
      4) Epidemiology: fecal-oral transmission of eggs, after ingestion, eggs hatch in the intestine, the larva penetrate the intestinal wall and enter the bloodstream, then the larva escape into the lungs, penetrate the alveoli and are coughed up the trachea

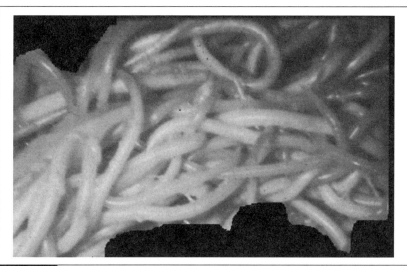

FIGURE 4.5 *Ascaris* **Worms**

Appearance of a mass of Ascaris *worms.*

so that they are swallowed back down into the intestine where they mature into adults and pass more eggs—**this is the most common parasitic infection in the world, with up to 1 billion people infected**

5) Clinical Diseases: although infection can be asymptomatic, **eosinophilic pneumonia** occurs during larval migration into the alveoli, malnutrition can occur due to adult worms scavenging nutrients in the gut, and **bowel obstruction** can occur due to luminal occlusion by large numbers of the large adult worms

6) Treatment: albendazole or mebendazole, pyrantel pamoate as 2nd line

7) Resistance: none

8) Prophylaxis: good hygiene

b. *Enterobius vermicularis* (pinworm)

1) Appearance: small white worms, 1 cm or less

2) Lab assays: scotch tape test = place scotch tape over anus and examine on a slide, the tape picks up the eggs which are visible under the microscope, worms can be directly visualized by stool O&P (but eggs are not present in stool)

3) Virulence factors: none significant

4) Epidemiology: **most common helminthic infection in the U.S.,** transmission is fecal-oral, **at night the female worm migrates out the anus and lays eggs in the perianal area**

5) Clinical Diseases: **perianal pruritus**

      6) Treatment: albendazole or mebendazole, pyrantel pamoate as 2nd line

      7) Resistance: none

      8) Prophylaxis: good hygiene

  c. Hookworm (*Ancylostoma duodenale* and *Necator americanus*)

      1) Appearance: long, thin worms, *Necator* has cutting plates to grab hold of the intestinal wall while *Ancylostoma* uses teeth

      2) Lab assays: stool O&P

      3) Virulence factors: none significant

      4) Epidemiology: **Ancylostoma duodenale is found in most of the underdeveloped world (Old World hookworm), while Necator americanus (New World hookworm) is found in the southeastern U.S., infection occurs via direct penetration of skin in contact with moist soil containing larvae,** like *Ascaris* the larvae migrate via blood to the lungs where they are coughed up and swallowed, allowing mature adults to develop in the intestines and to pass eggs in the stool

      5) Clinical Diseases: a pruritic, **erythematous dermatitis occurs at the site in the skin where the larvae penetrate, and eosinophilic pneumonia occurs** during transmigration of the larvae through the alveoli, some time after infection iron deficient anemia develops (**hookworm is the #1 cause of iron deficiency anemia in the world**), with all the usual anemia symptoms (e.g., weakness, fatigue, etc.), eosinophilia is typical

      6) Treatment: albendazole or mebendazole, pyrantel pamoate as 2nd line

      7) Resistance: none

      8) Prophylaxis: good sanitation, avoid direct skin contact with contaminated soil (e.g., don't walk barefoot through the soil)

  d. *Strongyloides stercoralis*

      1) Appearance: small round worms (see Figure 4.6)

      2) Lab assays: stool O&P

      3) Virulence factors: none significant

      4) Epidemiology: endemic throughout the tropical world, and also in the southeastern U.S., direct contact of skin with **soil contaminated by feces allows larval penetration into the host**, the larva migrates via blood to the lung where they are coughed up and swallowed, allowing adult maturation in the intestines, the adult worms lay eggs which either are defecated out to start the next cycle, or mature into larva within the infected host, allowing another round of infection within the same host in a process called autoinfection, **autoinfection can lead to overwhelming infection in immunocompromised patients**

      5) Clinical Diseases: **Cutaneous Larva Migrans = severe local contact dermatitis occurs at the site of skin penetration**, pts can be asymptomatic, but some develop diarrhea, eosinophilic

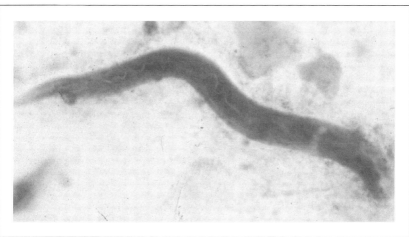

FIGURE 4.6 *Strongyloides*
Appearance of Strongyloides *in the sputum of an infected patient.*

pneumonia, or sepsis from bacterial translocation across a damaged gut wall, **peripheral eosinophilia is prominent**
6) Treatment: ivermectin or albendazole
7) Resistance: none
8) Prophylaxis: good sanitation, avoid bare skin contact with contaminated soil (e.g., don't walk barefoot through the soil)
e. *Trichuris trichiura* (whipworm)
1) Appearance: long thin worm, with a thread-like tail extending twice the length of the worm
2) Lab assays: stool O&P
3) Virulence factors: none significant
4) Epidemiology: fecal-oral transmission of eggs, eggs mature into adults in intestine, which then lay more eggs, there is no tissue phase
5) Clinical Diseases: often asymptomatic, but may cause invasive diarrhea, does NOT typically cause iron-deficient anemia, **in patients with heavy worm burden rectal prolapse can occur**
6) Treatment: albendazole or mebendazole
7) Resistance: none
8) Prophylaxis: good sanitation and good hygiene
f. *Trichinella spiralis*
1) Appearance: larvae are oval with ring-like centers, found in tissue, particularly muscle
2) Lab assays: **muscle biopsy, note stool O&P not helpful, look for marked eosinophilia**

3) Virulence factors: none significant
4) Epidemiology: typically transmitted via **ingestion of under-cooked pig, bear, or deer meat** containing larvae, larvae mature in the intestine, and lay eggs which penetrate into the bloodstream, seeding striated muscle throughout the body
5) Clinical Diseases: **Trichinosis**: an initial diarrhea is followed within 2 weeks by **severe myositis, headache with diffuse muscle aches, high fever, and extreme eosinophilia (up to 90% of peripheral white blood cells)**, can also cause CNS and cardiac damage
6) Treatment: albendazole or mebendazole with or without corticosteroids
7) Resistance: none
8) Prophylaxis: cook meats thoroughly

4. Tissue Roundworms (nematodes)
   a. *Dracunculus medinensis*
      1) Appearance: coiled worm up to a foot or more long can be seen burrowed beneath the skin, skin typically blisters and then ulcerates over the worm

TABLE 4.6	**Summary of Intestinal Roundworms (nematodes)**	
	TRANSMISSION	**CLINICAL Dz**
Ascaris	Fecal oral	Eosinophilic pneumonia, bowel obstruction
Enterobius	Fecal oral	Perianal pruritius in children
Ancylostoma	Skin penetration by larvae in moist soil	Pruritic, erythematosus dermatitis at site of penetration, iron deficient anemia and eosinophilia, occurs in Europe and Asia
Necator	Skin penetration by larvae in moist soil	Pruritic, erythematosus dermatitis at site of penetration, iron deficient anemia and eosinophilia, occurs in the SE U.S.
Strongyloides	Skin penetration by larvae in moist soil	Local contact dermatitis at site of skin penetration, diarrhea, eosinophilic pneumonia, sepsis
Trichuris	Fecal oral	Invasive diarrhea, rectal prolapse
Trichinella	Undercooked pork or game (bear or deer)	Diarrhea, severe myositis, headache, extreme eosinophilia

2) Lab assays: none
3) Virulence factors: none significant
4) Epidemiology: transmission is via **ingestion of fresh-water crustaceans containing larvae,** larvae mature in the intestine and the adult migrates to skin, the disease is on the decline in Africa due to WHO efforts to eradicate
5) Clinical Diseases: pruritic and painful welts overlying the sub-cutaneous worm, with ulceration over the worm's head
6) Treatment: surgical withdrawal of the worm
7) Resistance: none significant
8) Prophylaxis: boil or filter suspect drinking water, avoid ingestion

b. *Loa loa*
1) Appearance: can be seen as small (centimeter) subconjunctival worm burrowing across the eye or skin
2) Lab assays: thick and thin smear to identify parasites in the blood
3) Virulence factors: none significant
4) Epidemiology: endemic to Africa, transmitted by the bite of the deer fly
5) Clinical Diseases: **dermatitis or conjunctivitis caused by hyper-sensitivity to migrating worm in skin or eye**
6) Treatment: diethylcarbamazine, surgical excision may be required for conjunctival infections
7) Resistance: none
8) Prophylaxis: eradication of deer fly vector

c. *Oncocerca volvulus*
1) Appearance: worm less than a millimeter long
2) Lab assays: skin biopsy revealing the parasite
3) Virulence factors: none significant
4) Epidemiology: endemic to Africa, **particularly riverbeds, trans-mitted by bite of blackfly**, the organisms do not travel through blood, instead migrate subcutaneously
5) Clinical Diseases: **causes "river blindness"** (that's right, the people go blind from worm migration into the eyes, hence the name)
6) Treatment: ivermectin plus corticosteroids for patients with eye infection
7) Resistance: none
8) Prophylaxis: eradicate blackfly vector, ivermectin can be taken prophylactically

d. *Toxocara canis*
1) Appearance: not significant
2) Lab assays: tissue biopsy
3) Virulence factors: none significant

    4) Epidemiology: transmitted via **dog feces contaminating soil** and foodstuffs, eggs hatch into larvae in the intestine, the larvae then disseminate to multiple tissues

    5) Clinical Diseases: **"Visceral Larva Migrans" = diffuse granulomatous reactions causing fevers, myalgias, headache, CNS disease and retinal disease**, with a **prominent eosinophilia**, typically presents in children playing in soil with dogs

    6) Treatment: treat symptoms with corticosteroids and antihistamines, ivermectin, albendazole, or diethylcarbamazine for worms

    7) Resistance: none

    8) Prophylaxis: good sanitation and hygiene

  e. *Wuchereria bancrofti* and *Brugia malayi*

    1) Appearance: worm less than a millimeter long

    2) Lab assays: thick blood smears with blood drawn at night

    3) Virulence factors: none significant

    4) Epidemiology: ***Wuchereria* is endemic to Africa while *Brugia* is endemic to Asia** (particularly Malaysia hence the species name *malayi*), **both transmitted by mosquito bites,** organisms mature in lymph nodes and then circulate in the blood, particularly at night

    5) Clinical Diseases: **elephantiasis**, obstruction of lymphatics leads to severe lymphedema

    6) Treatment: ivermectin effective against larvae but not adult worms

    7) Resistance: none

    8) Prophylaxis: prevention of mosquito bites

TABLE 4.7	Summary of Invasive Roundworms (nematodes)	
	TRANSMISSION	**CLINICAL Dz**
Dracunculus	Freshwater crustaceans	Welts overlying the subcutaneous worm
Loa	Deerfly bite	Hypersensitivity to migrating worm
Oncocerca	Blackfly bite	Blindness
Toxocara	Dog feces	Visceral larva migrans = diffuse granulomas, retinitis, eosinophilia, headache, myalgias
Wuchereria and *Brugia*	Mosquito	Elephantiasis

TABLE 4.8	Overall Summary of Parasites	
	KEY WORD/PHRASE	**TREATMENT**
GI/GU Protozoa		
Cryptosporidium	• Diarrhea in AIDS patient	Immune reconstitution
Entamoeba	• Amoebic dysentery • Amoebic liver abscess	Metronidazole plus iodoquinol
Giardia	• Chronic non-bloody diarrhea in a hiker/camper	Metronidazole
Trichomonas	• Vaginitis with green, frothy discharge • Frequent recurrences because sexual partner needs treatment as well	Metronidazole
Invasive Protozoa		
Leishmania	• Sandfly bite in Asia, Africa, Latin America • Cutaneous ulcer • Lymphadenopathy, hepatosplenomegaly	Sodium stibogluconate
Plasmodium	• Mosquito bite in Africa, Mediterranean, Latin America • Shaking rigors, severe headache, myalgias • Cyclical fevers	Chloroquine ± primaquine
Toxoplasma	• Exposure to kitten feces or poorly cooked meat • Typically in AIDS pts with ring-enhancing brain lesions	Pyrimethamine + sulfadiazine + folinic acid
Trypanosoma	• Reduviid bug bite in Latin America • Tsetse fly bite in Africa • Romana's sign = swelling near eye where bite occurred • Heart block in young person Megacolon	Nifurtimox or suramin acutely, nothing works for chronic dz

(Continued)

TABLE 4.8	*Continued*	
	KEY WORD/PHRASE	**TREATMENT**
	Tapeworms (cestodes)	
Diphyllobothrium	• Raw fish consumption • B$_{12}$ deficiency	Albendazole
Echinococcus	• Shepherds, exposure to dogs and sheep • Large cysts seen in liver or lung	Albendazole and surgery
Hymenolepis	• Dog feces	Albendazole
Taenia saginata	• Undercooked beef • Tapeworm protrusion from anus	Albendazole
Taenia solium	• Undercooked pork or fecal-oral • Seizures and encephalitis in a Hispanic person	Albendazole ± seizure medicine
	Flukes (trematodes)	
Clonorchis	• Asian liver fluke • Raw freshwater fish	Albendazole
Paragonimus	• Asian lung fluke • Raw crab meat	Albendazole
Schistosoma	• Swimming in freshwater with snails nearby • Portal hypertension • Hematuria, bladder cancer	Albendazole
	Intestinal Roundworms (nematodes)	
Ascaris	• Eosinophilic pneumonia • Bowel obstruction • Iron deficiency	Albendazole
Enterobius	• Kid with itchy anus • Small white worms seen near anus • Eggs picked up from anus with scotch-tape	Albendazole

TABLE 4.8	*Continued*	
	KEY WORD/PHRASE	**TREATMENT**
Intestinal Roundworms (nematodes) (*Continued*)		
Ancylostoma	• Dermatitis at site of contact with moist soil • Iron deficiency anemia	Albendazole
Necator	• Dermatitis at site of contact with moist soil • Iron deficiency anemia • Southeastern U.S., poor areas	Albendazole
Strongyloides	• Local contact dermatitis (cutaneous larva migrans) at site of contact with moist soil • Eosinophilic pneumonia, auto infection	Ivermectin or albendazole
Trichuris	• Rectal prolapse	Albendazole
Trichinella	• Undercooked pig, bear, or deer meat • Severe myalgias with extreme eosinophilia	Albendazole
Invasive Roundworms (nematodes)		
Dracunculus	• Long worm seen coiled beneath soil	Worm extraction
Loa	• Small worm seen underneath conjunctiva	Diethylcarbamazine
Oncocerca	• Blackfly bite • River blindness in Africa	Ivermectin
Toxocara	• Visceral larva migrans • Retinal disease • Prominent eosinophilia	Steroids, antihistamines,? ivermectin
Wuchereria (Brugia)	• Elephantiasis	Ivermectin

V. VIRUSES

A. DNA Viruses

1. Naked DNA Viruses (unencapsulated)
   a. Adenovirus
      1) Genome: linear, double stranded DNA
      2) Lab assays: none significant
      3) Virulence factors: none significant
      4) Epidemiology: ubiquitous, airborne, fecal-oral, and fomite transmission, **outbreaks common in communal living situations,** e.g., military barracks
      5) Clinical Diseases: **mucosal infections,** including URIs, mild gastroenteritis, conjunctivitis, **classic illness is "pharyngoconjunctival fever,"** a combination conjunctivitis with pharyngitis
      6) Treatment: supportive
      7) Resistance: not applicable
      8) Prophylaxis: good hygiene, vaccine in use by the military
   b. Papovaviruses
      1) Human Papillomavirus (HPV)
         a) Genome: circular, double stranded DNA
         b) Lab assays: none significant
         c) Virulence factors: HPV E6 and E7 proteins are carcinogenic, inactivating p53 and the retinoblastoma (Rb) proto-oncogenes, respectively
         d) Epidemiology: ubiquitous, transmission by direct contact, especially through damaged skin
         e) Clinical Diseases:
            i)   HPV serotypes 1–4 cause common skin warts
            ii) HPV serotypes 6–11 cause genital warts
            iii) **HPV serotypes 16, 18, 31, 33, 35 cause cervical cancer, and are sexually transmitted**
         f) Treatment: freezing for skin warts, caustic application (e.g., podophyllin or salicylic acid) for genital warts, surgical excision with or without adjunctive radio- and chemotherapy for cervical cancer
         g) Resistance: not applicable
         h) Prophylaxis: good hygiene and safe sex
      2) Polyomaviruses: JC virus and BK virus
         a) Genome: circular, double stranded DNA
         b) Lab assays: none significant
         c) Virulence factors: none significant
         d) Epidemiology: affect immunocompromised, **JC seen in AIDS patients and BK seen in renal transplant patients**
         e) Clinical Diseases:

     i)   **JC Polyomavirus causes Progressive Multifocal Leukoencephalopathy in AIDS patients,** a relentlessly progressive encephalopathy which is almost invariably fatal

     ii) BK Polyomavirus causes severe nephritis in transplanted kidneys

  f) Treatment: immune reconstitution of AIDS patients for PML may lead to some benefit; cidofovir and reduction in immune suppression for renal transplant patients with BK virus (cidofovir tried for JC virus in PML with no conclusive benefit)

  g) Resistance: not applicable

  h) Prophylaxis: none

c. Parvovirus B19

  1) Genome: single stranded DNA

  2) Lab assays: serologies and PCR assay

  3) Virulence factors: none significant

  4) Epidemiology: ubiquitous, transmitted by contact, pregnant women should be isolated from infected patients due to the risk of transmission to the fetus

  5) Clinical Diseases:

    a) **Fifth Disease:** also known as erythema infectiosum or "slapped-cheek" disease, a mild viral exanthem seen in children causing **bright red erythema of the cheeks and lacy exanthem on the arms and trunk,** self-limiting

    b) **Aplastic anemia: Parvovirus B19 infection of chronic hemolysis pts** (e.g., Sickle Cell) can trigger aplastic crisis, **as the virus selectively infects stem cell precursors of RBCs,** particularly when stem cells are replicating quickly ($\uparrow$ replication during hemolysis as the body tries to repopulate RBCs)

    c) Hydrops fetalis: transplacental transmission can be lethal to the fetus

    d) Immune deposition arthritis develops in adults following URI

  6) Treatment: supportive; in immunocompromised patients (i.e., steroids or HIV) the aplastic anemia may be chronic and severe, and in these patients IVIG is of benefit to resolve the infection

  7) Resistance: not applicable

  8) Prophylaxis: good hygiene

2. Encapsulated DNA Viruses

  a. Hepadnavirus family

    1) Hepatitis B virus (HBV) (see Figure 5.1)

      a) Genome: circular, incompletely double stranded DNA

TABLE 5.1	Summary of Naked DNA Viruses	
VIRUS	**TRANSMISSION**	**DISEASE**
Adenovirus	Airborne, fecal-oral, & fomite	Conjunctivitis, pharyngitis, URI, gastroenteritis, classic dz is **pharyngoconjunctival fever**
HPV	Skin contact	Warts, cervical cancer
JC Polyomavirus	Unknown	Progressive Multifocal Leukoencephalopathy in AIDS
BK Polyomavirus	Unknown	Nephritis, renal graft rejection in transplant patients
Parvovirus B19	Contact	• 5th dz ("slapped cheek" viral exanthema) in kids • Aplastic anemia in chronic hemolysis patients • Hydrops fetalis in placental transmission to fetus • URI with arthritis in normal adults

b) Lab assays:
   i) **Hepatitis B surface antigen (HBsAg) levels in serum indicate active infection**
   ii) **Hepatitis B surface antibody (HBsAb) levels in serum indicate immunity to the virus**, during the development of immunity as the HBsAb titers rise, the surface antigen titers fall to undetectable
   iii) **Hepatitis B core antibody (HBcAb) levels in serum also indicate active infection, but they rise before surface antibody rises and are therefore positive in the window period when the surface antigen has fallen to undetectable but the surface antibody isn't yet detectable**
   iv) **The Hepatitis B e antigen (HBeAg) is expressed during viral replication, and is a marker for high risk of transmission due to active viral shedding**—being HBeAg positive carries a poor prognosis for rapid progression of disease
   v) Viral DNA levels in serum allow detection of active infection
c) Virulence factors: interesting life cycle, in which the virus transcribes its genome into mRNA and then uses reverse

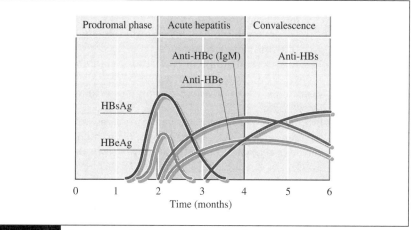

FIGURE 5.1 **Summary of Hepatitis B Serologies**

Time course of events following acute hepatitis B infection. (Reproduced by permission from Ayala C., Spellberg B. Boards and Wards. 2nd ed. Malden, MA: Blackwell Publishing, 2003: 33.)

transcriptase (of HIV fame) to generate a new DNA genome from the mRNA

d) Epidemiology: transmitted by body fluid contamination, most often via sexual transmission or IV drug abuse, but also via tattoo needles and blood transfusions (extremely rare now), but note that although rare in the U.S., **the #1 mode of transmission in the world is vertical, occurring in Asia where millions of infants are born with the virus**

e) Clinical Diseases:

  i)   Acute viral hepatitis with the usual fever, myalgias, nausea, vomiting, jaundice, transaminitis, the virus is cleared by 90% of patients

  ii) Chronic hepatitis: **10% of people who contract the disease as adults fail to clear the virus, but 90% of children who acquire the virus vertically fail to clear the virus,** leading to either an asymptomatic carrier state or chronic active hepatitis with nausea, vomiting, persistent transaminitis, immune-complex glomerulonephritis

  iii) Cirrhosis: occurs in patients with chronic active hepatitis

  iv) Hepatocellular carcinoma: develops in some people with chronic active hepatitis—**the risk of carcinoma is particularly high in children who acquire the disease** vertically, and hepatocellular carcinoma is one of the most common malignancies in the world because of the incredibly high prevalence in Asia where vertical transmission is common

   f) Treatment: lamivudine and/or adefovir (inhibitors of reverse transcriptase), or interferon-α

   g) Resistance: often develops during monotherapy with lamivudine

   h) Prophylaxis: the hepatitis B vaccine is a recombinant surface antigen with a >90% efficacy rate, recommended for health care workers, patients with underlying liver disease, drug abusers or anyone else at high risk for acquiring the virus

b. The Herpes Virus Family

  1) Herpes Simplex Virus-1 (HSV-1) (Human Herpes Virus 1)

    a) Genome: linear, double-stranded DNA

    b) Lab assays: Serology (not useful for diagnosing active disease), DFA, culture, Tzanck prep = scraping of base of an ulcer which on Wright–Giemsa stain reveals a clump of multinucleated giant cells, PCR of CSF

    c) Virulence factors: none significant

    d) Epidemiology: transmitted via saliva

    e) Clinical Diseases: typically causes cold sores, oral ulcers, conjunctivitis, and temporal lobe meningoencephalitis **(note these are all infections affecting the head)**

    f) Treatment: acyclovir

    g) Resistance: very rare

    h) Prophylaxis: good hygiene

  2) Herpes Simplex Virus-2 (HSV-2) (Human Herpes Virus 2)

    a) Genome: linear, double-stranded DNA

    b) Lab assays: Serology (not useful for diagnosing active disease), DFA, culture, Tzanck prep = scraping of base of an ulcer which on Wright–Giemsa stain reveals a clump of multinucleated giant cells

    c) Virulence factors: none significant

    d) Epidemiology: transmitted via sexual contact

    e) Clinical Diseases: typically causes vesicles that erode into **painful** ulcers (contrast with non-painful chancre of syphilis) on the genitals, can also cause oropharyngeal ulcers after oral sex, neonatal herpes can occur after transit of the infant through an infected vaginal canal, can also cause meningitis (a mild, often benign meningitis, in contrast with the deadly meningoencephalitis caused by HSV-1; HSV-2 may rarely also cause meningoencephalitis)

    f) Treatment: acyclovir

    g) Resistance: very rare

    h) Prophylaxis: safe sex

3) Varicella-Zoster Virus (VZV) (Human Herpes Virus 3)
   a) Genome: linear, double-stranded DNA
   b) Lab assays: PCR, serologies (not diagnostic of active infection), and Tzanck prep, but diagnosis is almost always clinical
   c) Virulence factors: **becomes latent in dorsal root ganglia**, allowing recrudescence after many years
   d) Epidemiology: transmitted is airborne
   e) Clinical Diseases:
      i) **Chicken pox**, a highly infectious childhood illness marked by classic, **pruritic, vesicular rash, appearing like a "dew-drop on a rose petal" with a central clearing on an erythematous macule**, immunity to first infection is usually lifelong so repeat episodes of chicken pox are rare—in chicken pox the lesions often start in the extremities and spread centrifugally to the trunk, the lesions form and mature at variable rates, so some will be newly forming as others vesicate and rupture, and others crust over
      ii) **Zoster, a reactivation disease usually seen in the immunocompromised or elderly, presents with a highly characteristic dermatomal vesicular rash and severe neuropathic pain along a dermatomal distribution, note that the pain can precede the rash by several days, so always think of Zoster if there is dermatomal pain even if no rash is apparent yet**
   f) Treatment: acyclovir
   g) Resistance: none
   h) Prophylaxis: vaccine is now available, recommended for all children and unexposed adults
4) Epstein-Barr Virus (EBV) (Human Herpes Virus 4)
   a) Genome: linear, double-stranded DNA
   b) Lab assays: **heterophile antibody (Monospot test)**; Epstein Bar Nuclear Antigen (EBNA), anti-viral core antibody (VCA)
   c) Virulence factors: binds to CD21 on B cells to initiate viral uptake
   d) Epidemiology: transmission is via saliva, >90% adults have been exposed
   e) Clinical Diseases:
      i) **Mononucleosis**, with fever, malaise, somnolence, and extensive lymphadenopathy with hepatosplenomegaly
      ii) EBV has been associated with Burkitt's lymphoma and non-Hodgkin's lymphoma, although causality has not been rigorously proven
      iii) Post-transplant lymphoproliferative disorder and CNS lymphoma in HIV patients are caused by EBV infection
   f) Treatment: none

g) Resistance: not applicable

h) Prophylaxis: none

5) Cytomegalovirus (CMV, Human Herpes Virus 5)

  a) Genome: linear, double-stranded DNA

  b) Lab assays: direct fluorescent antibody (DFA), serologies but >75% adults have positive titers so they may indicate prior exposure rather than active disease, serum buffy coat culture to detect viremia, DNA PCR of serum or body fluids (i.e., bronchoscopy wash) is the most useful test

  c) Virulence factors: none significant

  d) Epidemiology: transmitted by body fluid contamination, often via saliva or sexual transmission, also vertically and via organ transplants

  e) Clinical Diseases:

    i) Vertical transmission causes multiorgan disease, can be fatal to the fetus or infant, and is a common cause of mental retardation

    ii) Adult infection is often asymptomatic

    iii) **Viral syndrome indistinguishable from mononucleosis only heterophile antibody test is negative**

    iv) **Disseminated disease occurs in immunocompromised patients, can cause a granulomatous hepatitis, severe pneumonitis,** kidney disease, induce kidney graft rejection in transplant patients, and in AIDS patients causes diarrhea and vision threatening chorioretinitis

  f) Treatment: ganciclovir; more toxic alternatives include foscarnet and cidofovir

  g) Resistance: rare, except in transplant patients receiving prophylactic ganciclovir, in whom if CMV develops there is a reasonable chance of resistance requiring foscarnet or cidofovir

  h) Prophylaxis: good hygiene to avoid exposure

6) Human Herpes Virus 6 (HHV 6) & 7 (HHV 7)

  a) Genome: linear, double-stranded DNA

  b) Lab assays: none

  c) Epidemiology: probably transmitted via saliva

  d) Clinical Diseases: **Roseola infantum**, a childhood exanthem in which the child feels fine despite a high fever which lasts for up to 5 days, after the fever breaks a maculopapular rash erupts over the trunk and limbs and then resolves within about 24 hr; HHV 6 has been linked to severe organ disease in transplant patients

  e) Treatment: none

  f) Resistance: not applicable

  g) Prophylaxis: none

7) Human Herpes Virus 8 (HHV 8)

  a) Genome: linear, double-stranded DNA

  b) Lab assays: none

      c) Virulence factors: none significant
      d) Epidemiology: transmitted via sexual contact, particularly anoreceptive intercourse
      e) Clinical Diseases: **HHV 8 is accepted as the cause of Kaposi's sarcoma in AIDS patients** (i.e., epidemic Kaposi's), can also cause a much milder growth of endothelium seen in immunocompetent adults from the Mediterranean region (i.e., endemic Kaposi's), and is also strongly linked with Castleman's disease (multifocal lymphadenopathy, a low-grade pre-malignant condition)
      f) Treatment: immune reconstitution of HIV patients, chemoradiotherapy for Kaposi's Sarcoma, none for the virus
      g) Resistance: not applicable
      h) Prophylaxis: safe sex

  c. Poxviruses
    1) Molluscum contagiosum
      a) Genome: linear, double-stranded DNA
      b) Lab assays: biopsy
      c) Virulence factors: none significant
      d) Epidemiology: transmitted via direct contact with skin or fomites
      e) Clinical Disease: causes a classic papular rash, with papules that have pearly surface with **umbilicated center, can cause diffuse papules in AIDS patients**
      f) Treatment: liquid nitrogen freezing of papules
      g) Resistance: none
      h) Prophylaxis: good hygiene
    2) Monkeypox
      a) Genome: linear, double-stranded DNA
      b) Lab assays: PCR
      c) Virulence factors: none significant
      d) Epidemiology: transmitted via direct contact with skin or fomites from exotic pets, such as giant Gambian rats, cases in U.S. spread via exposed prairie dogs
      e) Clinical Disease: a pox rash
      f) Treatment: vaccination with the smallpox (vaccinia) vaccine post-exposure but prior to symptoms may abort clinical disease
      g) Resistance: none
      h) Prophylaxis: animal control efforts, smallpox (vaccinia) vaccine in certain cases
    3) Smallpox (Variola)
      a) Genome: linear, double-stranded DNA
      b) Lab assays: none
      c) Virulence factors: none significant
      d) Epidemiology: transmitted via direct contact with skin or fomites and by respiratory droplets, natural infection has been eradicated from the world, but several laboratories

around the world have frozen stocks and there is obviously the concern about bioterrorism

e) Clinical Disease:
   i) A chicken pox like diffuse papular-pustular rash, but in contrast to chicken pox it typically starts on face and trunk and spreads to extremities, and all lesions are in the same state at a given time (lesions form, umbilicate, and then crust together)
   ii) Disseminated disease with pneumonitis and sepsis (so-called flat smallpox)

f) Treatment: vaccination post-exposure but pre-symptoms can abort clinical disease; vaccinia immunoglobulin (VIG) can halt the spread of certain forms of smallpox

g) Resistance: none

h) Prophylaxis: vaccine was in widespread use in the U.S. until the early 1970s, the disease was eradicated globally in the 1970s, and vaccine use was then stopped and is now again being offered to select individuals (i.e., first responders, military etc.)—watch out for adverse events from the live virus vaccinia vaccine
   i) Progressive vaccinia occurs in patients with T cell deficiency (congenital or high dose steroids, theoretically in advanced AIDS but this hasn't been described) who receive the live virus vaccine, in which there is no inflammatory response to the vaccine but there is relentless, progressive necrosis at the vaccine site and then at disseminated locations, leading to extensive skin loss/tissue necrosis, superinfections, and shock—treat with VIG, ? cidofovir
   ii) Generalized vaccinia occurs in patients with mild immunodeficiencies, or with B cell deficiency, and may look very severe as the vaccine-induced papules can sprout all over the body, but this is rarely life-threatening—only treat with VIG if lesions are numerous
   iii) Vaccinia keratitis occurs due to auto-inoculation—treat with steroids, NOT VIG, which may cause antigen precipitation resulting in corneal clouding
   iv) Eczema vaccinatum—do not give the vaccinia vaccine to patients with eczema or atopic dermatitis; the vaccine will result in massive outbreak in such patients throughout the diseased skin, and can be fatal—treat with VIG
   v) Other adverse events have included encephalitis (rare) and myocarditis (common)—do not give the live virus vaccine to anyone with a known severe immunodeficiency (including HIV with CD4 count <200, however no evidence of adverse events if CD4 count >200), anyone with atopic dermatitis, or anyone with coronary disease as myocarditis may precipitate infarction

TABLE 5.2	Summary of Encapsulated DNA Viruses			
VIRUS	**TRANSMISSION**	**DISEASE**	**TREATMENT**	**VACCINE**
		Hepadnavirus		
HBV	Body fluids, vertical	Acute & chronic hepatitis, cirrhosis, hepatocellular carcinoma	Lamivudine/Adefovir	Yes
		Herpes Virus Family		
Cytomegalovirus	Body fluids, organ transplant, vertical	• Vertical transmission → mental retardation and death • Adults → asymptomatic or heterophile-negative mono • AIDS → diarrhea, hepatitis chorioretinitis, pneumonitis • Transplant pts → nephritis, hepatitis, pneumonitis	Ganciclovir	None
EBV	Saliva	Mononucleosis, ? lymphomas	Supportive	None
HSV-1	Saliva	Cold sores, conjunctivitis, meningoencephalitis	Acyclovir	None
HSV-2	Sexual	Genital vesicles and ulcers	Acyclovir	None

(Continued)

TABLE 5.2	*Continued*			
VIRUS	**TRANSMISSION**	**DISEASE**	**TREATMENT**	**VACCINE**
HHV 6 & 7	Saliva	Roseola infantum	None	None
HHV 8	Sexual	Kaposi's sarcoma	None	None
Varicella-Zoster	Airborne	Chicken pox, zoster	Acyclovir	Yes
Poxvirus				
Molluscum contagiosum	Skin contact	Skin papules with umbilicated centers	Mechanical removal	None
Monkeypox	Close contact	Febrile illness with ulcerating skin papules	None	Yes
Smallpox	Airborne or contact	Eradicated from world, caused papular rash and pneumonitis	None	Yes

B. RNA Viruses

1. Naked RNA Viruses (unencapsulated)
   a. Caliciviruses
      1) Hepatitis E Virus
         a) Genome: single-stranded RNA
         b) Lab assays: none significant
         c) Virulence factors: none significant
         d) Epidemiology: fecal-oral transmission
         e) Clinical Diseases: acute viral hepatitis much like hepatitis A virus; **however, note that hepatitis E virus causes high mortality in pregnant women**—this is a disease almost exclusively seen in non-industrialized countries
         f) Treatment: supportive
         g) Resistance: not applicable
         h) Prophylaxis: none
      2) Norwalk Virus
         a) Genome: single-stranded RNA
         b) Lab assays: none significant
         c) Virulence factors: none significant
         d) Epidemiology: fecal-oral transmission, **often via undercooked shellfish**
         e) Clinical Diseases: acute viral gastroenteritis, typically self-limited—this is the classic cause of gastroenteritis on cruise ships (look for cruise ships as buzzwords on the boards)
         f) Treatment: supportive
         g) Resistance: not applicable
         h) Prophylaxis: none
   b. Picornaviruses
      1) Enteroviruses (so-called because they are transmitted via the gastrointestinal, or "entero-," mucosa)
         a) Coxsackievirus
            i)   Genome: single-stranded RNA
            ii) Lab assays: none significant
            iii) Virulence factors: none significant
            iv) Epidemiology: fecal-oral and airborne transmission
            v)   Clinical Diseases:
                 a)) Aseptic meningitis: **one of the most common causes**
                 b)) Herpangina: pharyngitis with vesicles in posterior oropharynx
                 c)) Hand–Foot–Mouth dz: vesicles on hands and feet, with ulcers in oropharynx
                 d)) Myocarditis: a **dilated cardiomyopathy,** which can spontaneously resolve or can result in progressive congestive heart failure, causing death
                 e)) Serositis: pericarditis and pleuritis
                 f)) URI: mild flu-like illness

      vi) Treatment: supportive
      vii) Resistance: not applicable
      viii) Prophylaxis: none
  b) Echovirus
      i)   Genome: single-stranded RNA
      ii) Lab assays: none significant
      iii) Virulence factors: none significant
      iv) Epidemiology: fecal-oral transmission
      v) Clinical Diseases: **one of the most common causes of aseptic meningitis,** also URI
      vi) Treatment: supportive
      vii) Resistance: not applicable
      viii) Prophylaxis: none
  c) Hepatitis A Virus (HAV)
      i)   Genome: single-stranded RNA
      ii) Lab assays: serology
      iii) Virulence factors: none significant
      iv) Epidemiology: fecal-oral transmission
      v) Clinical Diseases: often asymptomatic, but in some pts causes acute viral hepatitis with fevers, abdominal pain, jaundice, dark urine, myalgias, transaminitis, very rare cause of fulminant hepatic failure
      vi) Treatment: supportive
      vii) Resistance: not applicable
      viii) Prophylaxis: an effective vaccine is available
  d) Poliovirus
      i)   Genome: single-stranded RNA
      ii) Lab assays: none significant
      iii) Virulence factors: **replicates in anterior horn motor neurons, causing neuronal death and paralysis**
      iv) Epidemiology: **fecal-oral transmission,** natural infection eradicated in the developed world—close to global eradication
      v) Clinical Diseases: **the vast majority of infections are totally asymptomatic, some people develop a flu-like viral syndrome which is self-limited, others develop meningitis, and some develop paralytic poliomyelitis,** note there is also a post-polio syndrome causing progressive myopathy and neuropathic pain, decades after initial clinical infection
      vi) Treatment: supportive
      vii) Resistance: not applicable
      viii) Prophylaxis:
          a)) Salk vaccine: an injectable killed poliovirus
          b)) Sabin vaccine: an oral attenuated virus
          c)) **Although Sabin used to be preferred, in the developed world it is no longer recommended due to**

TABLE 5.3	Summary of Naked RNA Viruses		
VIRUS	**TRANSMISSION**	**DISEASE**	**VACCINE**
Calicivirus (single-stranded RNA)			
Hepatitis E Virus	Fecal-oral	Acute viral hepatitis, note high mortality in pregnant women	None
Norwalk Virus	Fecal-oral	Acute viral gastro-enteritis, often after consumption of under-cooked shellfish, common on cruises	None
Picornavirus (single-stranded RNA)			
Enteroviruses			
Coxsackievirus	Fecal-oral, airborne	• Aseptic meningitis • Herpangina/Hand–Foot–Mouth disease • Myocarditis • Serositis • URI	None
Echovirus	Fecal-oral	Aseptic meningitis and URI	None
Hepatitis A Virus	Fecal-oral	Hepatitis	Yes
Poliovirus	Fecal-oral	Ranges from asymp-tomatic to URI to meningitis to paralytic polio, also post-polio degenerative disease	Yes (Sabin and Salk)
Rhinoviruses (single-stranded RNA)			
Rhinovirus	Airborne	Common cold	None
Reovirus Family (double-stranded RNA)			
Rotavirus	Fecal-oral	Diarrhea	None

the rare cases of polio from reversion of the vaccine to wild type—therefore the Salk vaccine is standard now, although Sabin may be used in developing countries

d)) **The Sabin vaccine should never be used for immunocompromised patients**

    2) Rhinovirus ("rhino-" = nose)
        a) Genome: single-stranded RNA
        b) Lab assays: none significant
        c) Virulence factors: binds to the ICAM-1 receptor on respiratory epithelium to mediate its uptake into human host, >100 serotypes makes vaccine development problematic
        d) Epidemiology: airborne transmission and fomites
        e) Clinical Diseases: **common cold**
        f) Treatment: supportive
        g) Resistance: not applicable
        h) Prophylaxis: good hygiene

  c. Reoviruses
    1) Rotavirus
        a) Genome: double-stranded RNA
        b) Lab assays: none significant
        c) Virulence factors: none significant
        d) Epidemiology: fecal-oral transmission
        e) Clinical Diseases: viral gastroenteritis, **Rotavirus is the most common cause of diarrhea worldwide,** usually affecting children ≤2 years old
        f) Treatment: supportive
        g) Resistance: not applicable
        h) Prophylaxis: good hygiene

2. Encapsulated RNA Viruses
  a. Positive RNA polarity (genomic RNA directly codes for protein)
    1) Coronaviruses
        a) coronavirus, multiple serotypes
          i)   Genome: single-stranded RNA
          ii) Lab assays: none
          iii) Virulence factors: none significant
          iv) Epidemiology: airborne
          v) Clinical Diseases: **common cold, 2nd most common cause behind Rhinoviruses**; also, a new coronavirus is the cause of the Severe Acute Respiratory Syndrome (SARS), acquired most likely from animals such as palm civets in Asia and then highly infectious spread from person to person by body fluid contact, fomites, and fecal-orally
          vi) Treatment: none
          vii) Resistance: not applicable
          viii) Prophylaxis: none
    2) Flaviviruses
        a) Dengue Virus
          i)   Genome: single-stranded RNA
          ii) Lab assays: none significant
          iii) Virulence factors: none significant

TABLE 5.4	Summary of Diagnostic Tests for Hepatitis Viruses	
VIRUS	**TEST**	**INTERPRETATION**
HAV	⊕IgM anti-HAV	Acute infection
	⊕IgG anti-HAV	Prior infection or vaccination—pt immune
HBV	⊕HBSAg	Patient is actively infected
	⊕HBSAb	Prior infection or vaccination (see below)—pt immune
	⊕HBCAb	Prior infection (NOT from vaccination)—pt may or may not be immune or actively infected (see below)
	⊕HBeAg	Pt is actively infected, rapid progression
	⊕HBV DNA viral load	Pt is actively infected
	⊕HBSAg, −HBCAb, −HBSAb	Acute infection (IgM CAb may be ⊕)
	−HBSAg, ⊕HBCAb, −HBSAb	Window period
	⊕HBSAg, ⊕HBCAb, −HBSAb	Chronic active infection
	−HBSAg, ⊕HBCAb, ⊕HBSAb	Prior infection, now immune
	−HBSAg, −HBCAb, ⊕HBSAb	Immune from vaccination, less likely prior infection with loss of HBCAb over time
HCV	⊕HCV Ab	Prior infection, 85% chance of chronic infection
	⊕HCV RNA	Active infection
	HCV genotype 1a	Poor response to Tx vs. all other genotypes
HDV	⊕HDV IgM	Suggest new infection

iv) Epidemiology: an arbovirus (transmitted by insect), transmitted by *Aedes* mosquito found in tropical areas, typical U.S. cases from tourists to the Caribbean

v) Clinical Diseases:

   a)) **Breakbone fever: severe flu-like syndrome, with unusually striking myalgias and arthralgias (pt feels like bones are breaking!),** rash is also common, although pt feels awful, breakbone fever is rarely fatal

   b)) **Dengue Hemorrhagic Fever:** starts like breakbone fever, but then diffuse mucosal hemorrhaging begins, typically from GI tract and skin, and shock ensues, frequently fatal—occurs in patients previously exposed to a different serotype of the Dengue virus

    vi) Treatment: supportive

    vii) Resistance: not applicable

    viii) Prophylaxis: insect repellent, avoid mosquitoes

b) Hepatitis C Virus (HCV)

    i) Genome: single-stranded RNA

    ii) Lab assays: serology, viral DNA levels in serum to detect active infection

    iii) Virulence factors: none significant

    iv) Epidemiology: transmitted via blood, by IVDA, needle-sticks, or blood transfusions, the possibility of sexual transmission is somewhat controversial

    v) Clinical Diseases: acute viral hepatitis, **up to 90% of people become chronically infected,** many of whom will end up with cirrhosis or hepatocellular carcinoma

    vi) Treatment: ribavirin and interferon-α, **a combination of the two has been proven to work better than either alone**

    vii) Resistance: serotype 1a is more resistant

    viii) Prophylaxis: avoid blood exposures, don't use drugs

c) Yellow Fever Virus

    i) Genome: single-stranded RNA

    ii) Lab assays: none

    iii) Virulence factors: none significant

    iv) Epidemiology: an arbovirus (transmitted by insect), transmitted by the *Aedes* mosquito found in tropical Africa and South America

    v) Clinical Diseases: **a severe viral syndrome causing hepatitis and which can progress to hemorrhagic fever,** often fatal

    vi) Treatment: none

    vii) Resistance: not applicable

    viii) Prophylaxis: avoid mosquitoes, a live-attenuated vaccine is available and is recommended for travelers to endemic areas

d) West Nile Virus

    i) Genome: single-stranded RNA

    ii) Lab assays: serology, PCR

    iii) Virulence factors: none significant

    iv) Epidemiology: an arbovirus transmitted by *Culex* mosquitoes, principally by spread through avian populations, and subsequently by biting people (dead end hosts)—initially spread to the U.S. in 1999, and has now spread across the entire U.S.

    v) Clinical disease: 80% of people are asymptomatically infected, 20% have a flu-like illness, <1% have full-blown encephalitis or meningitis often with severe sequelae or death

    vi) Treatment: supportive

    vii) Resistance: not applicable

    viii) Prophylaxis: avoid mosquitoes

3) Retroviruses

  a) Human Immunodeficiency Virus (HIV)

    i) Genome: single-stranded RNA, two copies per virus (diploid)

    ii) Lab assays:

      a)) **ELISA to screen for anti-HIV antibody**, 99.9% sensitive, 95% specific

      b)) **Western blot to confirm positive ELISA**, 95% sensitive, 99.9% specific

      c)) p24 antigen assay to directly detect virus in a patient who has not yet had time to develop antibody to the virus (can take up to 6 months)

      d)) Viral RNA can be directly quantified by PCR or by branched-DNA assays

      e)) CD4 T cell count to determine stage of disease (<200/μL = AIDS—please note that in the era of highly active antiretroviral therapy, the distinction between the terms HIV and AIDS has become almost irrelevant, as patients can be immune reconstituted from very low CD4 nadirs and AIDS is therefore no longer indicative of a short-term terminal condition)

    iii) Virulence factors:

      a)) **gp120** on the viral envelope **binds to CD4** and a 2nd co-receptor on T cells and other cells, the 2nd co-receptor is any of a number of chemokine receptors such as CCR5 and CXCR4

      b)) All retroviruses have *gag* genes coding for structural proteins, *pol* genes coding for reverse transcriptase, and *env* genes coding for viral envelop proteins

      c)) **HIV *gag* codes for a precursor to the p24 antigen** used clinically to detect infection during acute seroconversion syndrome, before patient's antibody response is positive—note that **protease inhibitors act against a viral protease which cleaves a large precursor viral protein into p24 and several other proteins**

      d)) **HIV *pol* protein codes for reverse transcriptase**

      e)) **HIV *env* protein codes for gp160**, which is spliced by a host protease into gp120 and gp41—note that protease inhibitors do NOT work against the protease which cleaves gp160, this is a host cell protease

f)) The mechanism of HIV-mediated destruction of CD4+ T cells is unclear; however, it probably relates to some combination of induction of CD8+ T-cell responses against HIV-infected CD4 cells, suppression of thymic selection of new T cells, direct CD4+ T-cell lysis, and exhaustion of bone marrow lymphocyte stem cells

iv) Epidemiology:

a)) Worldwide heterosexual and vertical transmission is the most common mode, in the U.S. homosexual transmission is still the most common and may be increasing again after a decade of decline; heterosexual transmission and IVDA transmission are increasing in the U.S.

b)) Africa has the most cases in the world now, but the most rapid spread is occurring in Southeast Asia and central Europe

c)) In the developed world, the death rate from AIDS has plummeted in the last 5 years, but it is not decreased in the underdeveloped world

d)) HIV has two major serotypes, HIV-1 and HIV-2, and dozens of clades, which are subtypes of HIV-1

e)) HIV-2 is virtually exclusively found in Western Africa, whereas HIV-1 is the dominant serotype found throughout the rest of the world

v) Clinical Disease:

a)) In most (>95%) patients AIDS is relentlessly progressive, and death occurs within 10 to 15 years of HIV infection

b)) Up to 5% of pts are "Long Term Survivors," meaning the disease does not progress even after 15 to 20 years without Tx—this may be due to infection with defective virus, a potent host immune response, or genetic resistance of the host, for example people with homozygous CCR5 deletions are highly resistant to HIV infection, and heterozygotes are less resistant

c)) Although patients can have no clinical evidence of disease for many years, HIV HAS NO LATENT PHASE; clinical silence in those patients who eventually progress is due to daily, temporarily successful host repopulation of T cells

d)) Death is usually caused by opportunistic infections (OIs) or malignancy

TABLE 5.5	CD4 Count and Opportunistic Infections	
CD4 COUNT	**DISEASE**	**PRIMARY PROPHYLAXIS**
Any	Tuberculosis: 10–100 fold ↑ risk	INH if PPD+
	Lymphoma: 10–100 fold ↑ risk	None
	Streptococcus pneumonia: 10–100 fold ↑ risk	Vaccinate
<200 cells/µL	*Pneumocystis*	Trimethoprim-sulfamethoxazole
	Kaposi's Sarcoma	None
<100 cells/µL	Toxoplasmosis	Trimethoprim-sulfamethoxazole
<50 cells/µL	*Mycobacterium avium intracellulare*	Azithromycin
	CMV	None
	Cryptosporidium	None
	CNS lymphoma	None

e)) Acute infection causes a mono-like seroconversion syndrome with rash, fevers, lymphadenopathy, transaminitis, and sometimes meningitis
f)) Then an asymptomatic phase sets in for several years while CD4+ T-cells are steadily destroyed
g)) As T cells fall below 200, the patient becomes susceptible to opportunistic infections and malignancies
vi) Treatment:
a)) Highly Active Antiretroviral Therapy (HAART): **all patients with HIV should be receiving three or more drugs at a time**, including some combination of a viral nucleoside analogue, a protease inhibitor, and/or a non-nucleoside reverse transcriptase inhibitor; entry inhibitors (e.g., fuzeon) are now available
b)) The overall success of HAART is about 60–80% at reducing the viral load below the limit of detectability, and the principle cause of HAART-failure is non-compliance
c)) **All HIV⊕ patients with CD4 counts <200/µL should be on trimethoprim-sulfamethoxazole prophylaxis for *Pneumocystis* pneumonia (PCP) and *Toxoplasma***

        d)) **All HIV⊕ patients with CD4 counts <50/μL should be on azithromycin prophylaxis for** *Mycobacterium avium intracellulare* **infection**

        e)) Resistance: **invariable if treated with less than three drugs, and will occur despite any regimen if compliance is poor**

        f)) Prophylaxis: avoid unprotected sex, sharing needles, and needle-sticks, avoid mucosal splashes with body secretions

  b) Human T-cell Leukemia Virus (HTLV)

    i) Genome: single-stranded RNA

    ii) Lab assays: serology

    iii) Virulence factors: ability to integrate into host DNA causing cellular transformation

    iv) Epidemiology: transmitted via blood-products and unsafe sex, **HTLV is most prevalent in Japan and in the Caribbean**, there are two dominant serotypes, HTLV-1 and HTLV-2

    v) Clinical Diseases:

        a)) Human T cell leukemia and cutaneous T cell lymphomas

        b)) **Tropical spastic paraparesis**: a condition of **degeneration of spinal motor neurons leading to hyperspasticity and paresthesias** of the lower extremities accompanied by incontinence of urine and neuropathic pain

    vi) Treatment: none

    vii) Resistance: not applicable

    viii) Prophylaxis: avoid exposure to blood-products and unsafe sex

4) Togaviruses

  a) Encephalitis Viruses

    i) Genome: single-stranded RNA

    ii) Lab assays: serology, CSF culture

    iii) Virulence factors: none significant

    iv) Epidemiology:

        a)) All are arboviruses ("arthropod-borne") transmitted by mosquitoes, with wild birds acting as normal hosts

        b)) Eastern Equine Encephalitis Virus is the most severe, with a case fatality rate approaching 50%

        c)) Western Equine Encephalitis Virus causes less severe infections

        d)) St. Louis Encephalitis Virus has a case fatality rate between Eastern and Western Equine Viruses

    v) Clinical Diseases: encephalitis which is often fatal in the young or elderly

  vi) Treatment: supportive
  vii) Resistance: not applicable
  viii) Prophylaxis: avoid mosquitoes
 b) Rubella
  i) Genome: single-stranded RNA
  ii) Lab assays: serology, CSF culture
  iii) Virulence factors: none significant
  iv) Epidemiology: airborne transmission, can be transplacentally transmitted
  v) Clinical Diseases: transplacental transmission causes congenital cardiac, neurological, and ocular malformations, **childhood infection causes the German measles, with a fever and maculopapular rash which is self-limiting**
  vi) Treatment: supportive
  vii) Resistance: not applicable
  viii) Prophylaxis: live-attenuated vaccine
 b. Negative RNA polarity (genomic RNA must be transcribed into a complementary strand which codes for protein, thus these viruses require their own RNA polymerase)
  1) Arenaviruses
   a) Lymphocytic Choriomeningitis (LCM) Virus
    i) Genome: single-stranded RNA
    ii) Lab assays: none significant
    iii) Virulence factors: none significant
    iv) Epidemiology: exact mode of transmission unclear, but **exposure to house mice or other rodents is a requisite**
    v) Clinical Diseases: a flu-like illness with rash and leukopenia which can within days progress to **aseptic meningitis of unusual severity, and which may be fatal**
    vi) Treatment: supportive
    vii) Resistance: not applicable
    viii) Prophylaxis: avoid rodents
   b) Lassa Fever Virus
    i) Genome: single-stranded RNA
    ii) Lab assays: none significant
    iii) Virulence factors: none significant
    iv) Epidemiology: exact mode of transmission unclear, but exposure to rodents and direct human contact are involved, most cases occur in West Africa
    v) Clinical Diseases: a flu-like illness that can progress to cause disseminated disease, including cranial nerve deficits, hepatitis, and **microcapillary leak leading to hemorrhagic fever and shock**
    vi) Treatment: supportive
    vii) Resistance: not applicable
    viii) Prophylaxis: avoid rodents

2) Bunyaviruses
   a) California Encephalitis Virus
      i) Genome: single-stranded RNA
      ii) Lab assays: serology
      iii) Virulence factors: none significant
      iv) Epidemiology: an arbovirus, spread by mosquitoes, actually occurs over much of North America
      v) Clinical Diseases: encephalitis, typically in children and teens
      vi) Treatment: supportive
      vii) Resistance: not applicable
      viii) Prophylaxis: avoid mosquitoes
   b) Hantavirus
      i) Genome: single-stranded RNA
      ii) Lab assays: serology
      iii) Virulence factors: none significant
      iv) Epidemiology: **spread by inhalation of dust particles from house mice feces, cases typically reported in desert areas like Nevada, New Mexico, and Arizona,** exposure typically in rural area the summer after a wet spring when the rodent population increases
      v) Clinical Diseases: **a flu-like illness which can rapidly progress in hours to acute respiratory distress syndrome (ARDS),** and has a fatality rate of >50%
      vi) Treatment: supportive
      vii) Resistance: not applicable
      viii) Prophylaxis: rodent population control
3) Deltavirus
   a) Hepatitis D Virus (HDV)
      i) Genome: single-stranded RNA
      ii) Lab assays: serology
      iii) Virulence factors: none significant
      iv) Epidemiology: transmitted by body fluids, typically IVDA or sex, the virus is defective and **cannot replicate unless Hepatitis B Virus co-infects the same cell,** in which case HDV can use proteins made by HBV to replicate
      v) Clinical Diseases: **simultaneous infection of HBV and HDV leads to an acute hepatitis** somewhat more severe than HBV infection alone; **however, if a person is already infected with HBV and then gets HDV on top, it can cause a very severe hepatitis which can progress to fulminant hepatic failure**
      vi) Treatment: supportive
      vii) Resistance: not applicable
      viii) Prophylaxis: safe sex, don't use drugs, immunization with HBV vaccine

4) Filoviruses
   a) Ebola & Marburg Viruses
      i) Genome: single-stranded RNA
      ii) Lab assays: serology
      iii) Virulence factors: none significant
      iv) Epidemiology: mode of transmission not entirely clear, seems to be direct contact with blood or infected meat from primates in Africa; how commonly human to human transmission occurs is not clear
      v) Clinical Diseases: **flu-like illness progresses to hemorrhagic fever,** with microangiopathic capillary destruction and bleeding from every orifice, causing circulatory collapse, a frighteningly **high mortality rate approaching 80–90%**
      vi) Treatment: supportive, immune serum from convalescing patients has been transfused to newly infected patients during outbreaks, but efficacy is not established
      vii) Resistance: not applicable
      viii) Prophylaxis: none
5) Orthomyxoviruses
   a) Influenza
      i) Genome: segmented, single-stranded RNA (unlike Paramyxoviruses which have single piece of RNA, Orthomyxoviruses have their RNA chopped up into segments, Influenza has eight of these segments)
      ii) Lab assays: culture, rapid influenza ELISA
      iii) Virulence factors:
         a)) **Hemagglutinin binds to host cells to mediate uptake** and **neuraminidase cleaves the virus free of the membrane** to allow the virus to enter the cytoplasm of the infected cell
         b)) **Antigenic drift** is the **progressive, steady mutation of the hemagglutinin and neuraminidase** which allows the virus to come back each year with a slightly different structure so that prior acquired immunity is less effective
         c)) **Antigenic shift is due to sudden genetic recombination of hemagglutinin and neuraminidase with other influenza types, causing instant generation of brand new viral strains**
         d)) Antigenic shift totally negates the effect of prior immunity, since a wholly new virus is created which no immune system has ever seen, and this is responsible for periodic pandemics which can kill millions across the globe every few decades

e)) There are also three serotypes of Influenza, called Types A, B, and C, with **A being the most common etiologic agent of human disease**

iv) Epidemiology: airborne transmission, new viral strains are typically generated in Asia and then spread west across the globe

v) Clinical Diseases: Influenza is different than the common cold, with **high fever, striking myalgias** (particularly of the long muscles in the back and in the hamstrings), cough and headache, **but vomiting, diarrhea, and rhinorrhea are typically NOT present,** in elderly patients secondary **bacterial infections can set in during the resolution phase of Influenza infections, causing a biphasic presentation** of severe illness, followed by recovery, followed by sudden decompensation with cough newly productive of purulent sputum

vi) Treatment:

a)) Neuraminidase inhibitors (oseltamivir and zanamivir) are effective at decreasing the severity of Influenza A and B infections and shortening their duration by a day or two if started within 48 hrs of onset of symptoms

b)) Amantadine and rimantadine are only active against Influenza A and also must be started within 48 hrs of symptoms to be effective

vii) Resistance: described for amantadine and rimantadine, very rare for neuraminidase inhibitors

viii) Prophylaxis:

a)) Killed vaccine contains mixture of Influenza A & B and **is reformulated every year based on serotypes causing disease each year, but protection lasts <1 yr so yearly revaccination required**

b)) Vaccine recommended for: pts >50 yrs old (new rec as of 2000), pts with co-morbid dz (e.g., heart, lung, liver, kidney dz, diabetes, cancer), close contacts of such people, **and health care workers**

c)) A live-attenuated inhaled vaccine is now available

d)) Amantadine can prevent Influenza A (but not B), useful for elderly contacts of pts with the flu

6) Paramyxoviruses

a) Measles Virus

i) Genome: single-stranded RNA

ii) Lab assays: serology

iii) Virulence factors: none significant

iv) Epidemiology: airborne transmission

v) Clinical Diseases: **childhood exanthem with a classic 3 Cs of cough, coryza, and conjunctivitis, along with** maculopapular rash which starts on the face and migrates down to the trunk, Koplik's spots are red macules with a white center found on the buccal mucosa, but while these are pathognomonic they occur prior to the onset of the rash and typically resolve prior to the onset of the rash, so **they are often not present when the child presents**, note that measles can be life-threatening in immunocompromised children

   vi) Treatment: supportive

   vii) Resistance: not applicable

   viii) Prophylaxis: a highly effective live-attenuated vaccine

b) Mumps Virus

   i) Genome: single-stranded RNA

   ii) Lab assays: serology

   iii) Virulence factors: none significant

   iv) Epidemiology: airborne transmission

   v) Clinical Diseases: **flu-like prodrome leads in to acute onset of parotid swelling** (unilateral or bilateral), although typically self-limiting after a week or so, **some post-pubescent males can develop orchitis which can cause sterility if bilateral**, and rarely patients may develop aseptic meningitis

   vi) Treatment: supportive

   vii) Resistance: not applicable

   viii) Prophylaxis: a highly effective live-attenuated vaccine

c) Parainfluenza Virus

   i) Genome: single-stranded RNA

   ii) Lab assays: none significant

   iii) Virulence factors: none significant

   iv) Epidemiology: airborne transmission

   v) Clinical Diseases: presents in **children with Croup, a laryngotracheobronchitis typified by a dry, "barking cough"** and hoarse voice, can cause any URI in adults

   vi) Treatment: supportive, inhaled bronchodilators and inhaled, humidified air are helpful measures in patients with Croup

   vii) Resistance: not applicable

   viii) Prophylaxis: none

d) Respiratory Syncytial Virus (RSV)

   i) Genome: single-stranded RNA

   ii) Lab assays: Direct Fluorescent Antibody

   iii) Virulence factors: none significant

   iv) Epidemiology: airborne transmission

   v) Clinical Diseases: mild URI in older children and adults, but can cause a **severe pneumonia in young children**, is a common cause of acute respiratory distress syndrome in them

TABLE 5.6	**Summary of Encapsulated RNA Viruses**		
VIRUS	**TRANSMISSION**	**DISEASE**	**VACCINE**
Coronavirus (positive polarity)			
Coronavirus	Airborne	Common cold or SARS	None
Flaviviruses (positive polarity)			
Dengue Virus	*Aedes* mosquito	Breakbone & hemorrhagic fever	None
Hepatitis C Virus	Blood	Hepatitis, cirrhosis, hepatocellular CA	None
Yellow Fever	*Aedes* mosquito	Hepatitis, hemorrhagic fever	Yes
West Nile Virus	*Culex* mosquito	Asymptomatic or meningoencephalitis	No
Retroviruses (positive polarity)			
HIV	Body fluids, sex	Acute seroconversion syndrome, AIDS	No
HTLV	Body fluids, sex	T-cell leukemia/ lymphoma and tropical spastic paraparesis, common in Japan and the Caribbean	No
Togaviruses (positive polarity)			
Encephalitis Viruses	Mosquito bite	Encephalitis	No
Rubella	Airborne, vertical	German measles, congenital defects	Yes
Arenaviruses (negative polarity)			
LCM Virus	Rodent exposure	Severe aseptic meningitis	No
Lassa Fever Virus	Rodent exposure	Hemorrhagic fever	No
Bunyaviruses (negative polarity)			
California Encephalitis Virus	Mosquitoes	Encephalitis	No
Hantavirus	Rodent droppings	ARDS	No

TABLE 5.6 *Continued*			
VIRUS	**TRANSMISSION**	**DISEASE**	**VACCINE**
Deltavirus (negative polarity)			
Hepatitis D Virus	Body fluids, sex	Hepatitis (in conjunction with HBV)	Yes*
Filoviruses (negative polarity)			
Ebola-Marburg	Unknown	Hemorrhagic fever	No
Orthomyxoviruses (negative polarity)			
Influenza	Airborne	The flu	Yes
Paramyxoviruses (negative polarity)			
Measles	Airborne	Measles: cough, coryza, conjunctivitis	Yes
Mumps	Airborne	Mumps: parotid swelling, orchitis	Yes
Parainfluenza Virus	Airborne	Croup: barking cough	No
Respiratory Syncytial Virus	Airborne	URI in older kids, pneumonia in younger	No
Rhabdovirus (negative polarity)			
Rabies Virus	Animal bite	Confusion, hydrophobia, seizures, coma	Yes

* The HBV vaccine is effective against HDV because HBV is necessary for HDV to cause disease.

      vi) Treatment: ribavirin is used, but efficacy unclear
      vii) Resistance: not applicable
      viii) Prophylaxis: none
  7) Rhabdovirus
    a) Rabies Virus
      i) Genome: single-stranded RNA
      ii) Lab assays: **biopsy of infected neurons showing Negri bodies**
      iii) Virulence factors: binds to the acetylcholine receptor to mediate uptake into neurons
      iv) Epidemiology:
        a)) **Transmitted via saliva into bite by rabid animal**, cases are exceedingly rare in the U.S. due to frequent vaccination of animals, but the **virus is**

TABLE 5.7	**Overall Summary of Viruses**		
	GENOME	**KEY WORD/PHRASES**	**VACCINE**
		Naked DNA Viruses	
Adenovirus	dsDNA	Pharyngoconjunctival fever, gastroenteritis	No
Human Papillomavirus	dsDNA	Warts, cervical cancer, fomite transmission	No
JC Polyomavirus	dsDNA	Encephalopathy (PML) in AIDS pts	No
BK Polyomavirus	dsDNA	Nephritis in kidney transplants	No
Parvovirus B19	ssDNA	Aplastic crisis in hemolysis pts, 5th dz in kids	No
		Encapsulated DNA Viruses	
Hepatitis B Virus	dsDNA	10% of adults get chronic infection, 90% of vertically transmitted is chronic, tx with lamivudine, adefovir, or interferon-α	Yes
Cytomegalovirus	dsDNA	HHV 5, heterophile-negative mononucleosis in healthy people, severe hepatitis, pneumonia, retinitis in AIDS or organ transplant patients	No
Epstein-Barr Virus	dsDNA	HHV 4, heterophile-positive mononucleosis	No
Herpes Simplex 1	dsDNA	HHV 1, oral ulcers, conjunctivitis, meningitis	No
Herpes Simplex 2	dsDNA	HHV 2, genital ulcers, meningitis	No
HHV 6 & 7	dsDNA	Roseola infantum	No
HHV 8	dsDNA	Kaposi's sarcoma in AIDS pts	No
Varicella-Zoster Virus	dsDNA	HHV 3, chicken pox and zoster (dermatomal pain and vesicular rash in elderly and sick)	Yes
Molluscum Poxvirus	dsDNA	Molluscum contagiosum in AIDS pts	No
Smallpox	dsDNA	Smallpox, eradicated from globe	Yes
Monkeypox	dsDNA	Exotic pet exposure	Yes*

TABLE 5.7 *Continued*			
	GENOME	**KEY WORD/PHRASES**	**VACCINE**
Naked RNA Viruses			
Hepatitis E	ss⊕ RNA	Hepatitis with high mortality in pregnancy	No
Norwalk	ss⊕ RNA	Gastroenteritis, often undercooked shellfish	No
Coxsackievirus	ss⊕ RNA	An enterovirus, causes multiple diseases including URI, serositis, myocarditis, Hand–Foot–Mouth dz, Herpangina, and meningitis	No
Echovirus	ss⊕ RNA	An enterovirus, causes URI and meningitis	No
Hepatitis A	ss⊕ RNA	Acute viral hepatitis	Yes
Polio	ss⊕ RNA	Rare pts get meningitis and full-blown polio	Yes
Rhinovirus	ss⊕ RNA	#1 cause of the common cold	No
Rotavirus	dsRNA	#1 cause diarrhea in the world, often age <2	No
Encapsulated RNA Viruses			
Coronavirus	ss⊕ RNA	Common cold or SARS	No
Dengue	ss⊕ RNA	Breakbone fever (myalgias and arthralgias so severe it feels like bones are breaking)	No
Hepatitis C	ss⊕ RNA	90% of infected have chronic dz, treat with combination ribavirin and interferon-α	No
Yellow Fever	ss⊕ RNA	Severe hepatitis and hemorrhagic fever	Yes
West Nile	ss⊕ RNA	Mosquito-born meningoen-cephalitis in humans and birds	No
Human Immunodeficiency	ss⊕ RNA	P24 antigen present during seroconversion when ELISA is negative, kills CD4 T cells, death from infection or malignancy	No
Human T-cell Leukemia	ss⊕ RNA	Causes T-cell leukemia and lymphoma, and tropical spastic paraparesis, highest prevalence in Japan and the Caribbean	No

(Continued)

TABLE 5.7	*Continued*		
	GENOME	**KEY WORD/PHRASES**	**VACCINE**
Encephalitis	ss⊕ RNA	Transmitted by mosquitoes, often fatal	No
Rubella	ss⊕ RNA	German measles = fever and rash, self-lmtd	Yes
Lymphocytic Choriomeningitis	ss– RNA	Severe aseptic meningitis, may be fatal	No
Lassa Fever	ss– RNA	Hemorrhagic fever	No
California Encephalitis	ss– RNA	Transmitted by mosquito	No
Hantavirus	ss– RNA	Exposure to rodents in rural desert areas, causes rapidly progressive ARDS	No
Hepatitis D	ss– RNA	Only infective in the presence of HBV	Yes†
Ebola-Marburg	ss– RNA	Hemorrhagic fever, up to 90% mortality	No
Influenza	ss– RNA	Striking myalgias and fever, no GI symptoms	Yes
Measles	ss– RNA	Cough, coryza, conjunctivitis, maculopapular rash, Koplick's spots	Yes
Mumps	ss– RNA	Rash, parotid swelling, orchitis	Yes
Parainfluenza	ss– RNA	Croup, hoarse voice and "barking cough"	No
Respiratory Syncytial	ss– RNA	URI in older kids, pneumonia in younger kids	No
Rabies	ss– RNA	Binds to acetylcholine receptor, migrates to CNS so bites closer to head cause disease more rapidly, classic symptom is hydrophobia where pt fears drinking water due to painful spasms in oropharynx when swallowing	Yes

* Smallpox vaccine provides partial protection against Monkeypox.

† For HDV, the HBV vaccine is effective since HDV only causes dz in the presence of HBV.

ds, double-stranded; ss, single-stranded; ⊕, positive polarity; –, negative polarity; HHV, Human Herpes Virus.

common in bats and skunks throughout the U.S. and can occur in **canines near the U.S.–Mexico border**

b)) Following inoculation in the wound, the virus binds to peripheral neurons and is carried retrograde back to the CNS where it infects parts of the brain controlling aggression, making infected individuals prone to biting which can spread the virus to a new host

v) Clinical Diseases: within several weeks of bite (shorter time the closer the bite is to the head) the patient develops flu-like prodrome followed by acute onset of altered mental status, hypersalivation, and **painful spasms in the oropharynx on swallowing leading to the classic symptom of hydrophobia where a patient is afraid to swallow water due to the pain,** the disease inevitably progresses from seizures to coma, death is invariable

vi) Treatment: supportive once disease onsets

vii) Resistance: not applicable

viii) Prophylaxis:

a)) Pre-exposure prophylaxis is via rabies vaccine, which should be given to anyone in contact with wild animals

b)) **Post-exposure prophylaxis is via both administration of rabies vaccine and rabies immune globulin given concurrently but at different sites to prevent neutralization of the vaccine by the antibody**

VI. ANTIBIOTICS

A. Bacterial Agents

1. Penicillins
   a. Mechanism: **inhibits bacterial cell wall synthesis** by blocking the **transpeptidase**-dependent cross-linkage of peptidoglycan
   b. Resistance: several mechanisms described
      1) **β-lactamase production**: many bacteria express β-lactamase, an enzyme that cleaves open the 4-membered β-lactam ring in penicillins, inactivating them—this can be overcome by adding a β-lactamase inhibitor to the penicillin, which protects the penicillin from the bacterial β-lactamase
      2) Altered penicillin binding proteins (PBPs): some bacteria have mutated penicillin binding targets (the transpeptidases), this is the mechanism for Methicillin-Resistant *Staphylococcus aureus* (MRSA)
   c. Toxicities: hypersensitivity reactions (including anaphylaxis) common, can also see leukopenia and can induce autoimmune hemolytic anemia
   d. Cidal/Static: cidal for actively dividing bacteria
   e. Coverage:
      1) Penicillin: good *Strep* coverage and **good for oral anaerobes**, good for strep throat, oral/dental infections, syphilis, bad for gram negatives
      2) Aminopenicillins (e.g., ampicillin): addition of amino group **adds coverage for *Enterococcus* and *Listeria***, and some gram negatives
      3) Addition of β-lactamase inhibitor (e.g., ampicillin + sulbactam): **markedly expands coverage**, including most *Enterococcus*, *Staphylococcus* (not MRSA), most *Streptococcus*, most community acquired gram negative rods (but not nosocomials like *Pseudomonas*), most anaerobes (including abdominal anaerobes)
      4) Penicillinase-resistant penicillins (e.g., oxacillin): **specifically designed to hit *Staphylococcus***, covers all *Staphylococcus* except those with altered penicillin binding proteins (so-called Methicillin Resistant Staphylococci or MRSA) at the expense of losing some coverage on *Streptococcus* and losing all coverage on *Enterococcus* and gram negatives
      5) Ureidopenicillins (e.g., piperacillin): **designed for expanded gram negative coverage**, covers gram positives per aminopenicillins, but **also covers nosocomial gram negatives** like many strains of *Pseudomonas*—note that **addition of β-lactamase inhibitor (e.g., piperacillin/tazobactam)**

creates an incredibly powerful drug which covers virtually all gram positives (except MRSA and some *Enterococcus*), virtually all gram negatives including most *Pseudomonas*, and virtually all anaerobes

2. Cephalosporins
   a. Mechanism: like penicillins, **inhibits bacterial cell wall synthesis** by blocking the transpeptidase-dependent cross-linkage of peptidoglycan
   b. Resistance: two major mechanisms
      1) β-lactamase production: although cephalosporins have a 6-membered ring instead of the 4-membered β-lactam ring, β-lactamase enzymes still destroy cephalosporins
      2) Altered penicillin binding proteins
   c. Toxicities: hypersensitivity reactions less common than penicillins and **only 15% cross-reactivity between penicillin allergy and cephalosporin allergy**, cephalosporins also can cause biliary sludging, and cause coagulation abnormalities due to vitamin K depletion
   d. Cidal/Static: cidal for actively dividing bacteria
   e. Coverage:
      1) 1st generation (e.g., cefazolin): very good *Staphylococcus* and *Streptococcus* coverage, makes them **good for skin infections**, and hits community acquired gram negatives (e.g., *E. coli*) so good for UTIs
      2) 2nd generation (e.g., cefuroxime): better *Streptococcus* coverage but worse *Staphylococcus* coverage, better community acquired gram negative coverage, **good for outpatient community acquired pneumonia**, some have very good anaerobic coverage (e.g., cefotetan)
      3) 3rd generation: difficult to assess by class, two specifics to know
         a) Ceftriaxone: **best *Streptococcus* coverage of all, loses most *Staphylococcus* coverage, good community acquired gram negatives but does not hit nosocomial gram negatives,** 1st line for meningitis and in-patient community acquired pneumonia
         b) Ceftazidime: **loses all gram positive coverage but excellent gram negative coverage including most nosocomials including *Pseudomonas*, used for nosocomial infections**

3. Carbapenems
   a. Mechanism: like penicillins, inhibits bacterial cell wall synthesis by blocking the transpeptidase-dependent cross-linkage of peptidoglycan

     b. Resistance: most β-lactamases don't work well against carbapenems so this is a rare (but increasing) mechanism of resistance, however altered penicillin binding proteins still a problem

     c. Toxicities: seizures

     d. Cidal/Static: cidal for actively dividing bacteria

     e. Coverage: imipenem and meropenem are very similar except meropenem may less frequently cause seizures, both probably the broadest spectrum coverage available in any one drug, cover most gram positives, most gram negatives including *Pseudomonas*, and most anaerobes

4. Monobactams

     a. Mechanism: like penicillins, inhibits bacterial cell wall synthesis by blocking the transpeptidase-dependent cross-linkage of peptidoglycan

     b. Resistance: β-lactamases don't work well against monobactams so this is not a mechanism of resistance, however altered penicillin binding proteins still a problem

     c. Toxicities: minimal, no cross-reactivity to penicillins

     d. Cidal/Static: cidal for actively dividing bacteria

     e. Coverage: one drug, aztreonam, **covers most gram negatives including nosocomials like *Pseudomonas*, but loses all anaerobic and gram positive coverage**

5. Glycopeptide

     a. Mechanism: like penicillins, **inhibits bacterial cell wall synthesis,** but unlike penicillins they **act by binding to D-alanine-D-alanine subunits of the cell wall** and preventing their insertion into the cell wall

     b. Resistance: all gram negatives are intrinsically resistant, gram positive resistance is unusual but can occur via a variety of mechanisms

     c. Toxicities: azotemia, "Red Man syndrome" (skin flushing)

     d. Cidal/Static: static

     e. Coverage: vancomycin is the major parenteral version (teicoplanin is not yet approved in the U.S.), bacitracin is a topical version, vancomycin **covers all gram positive organisms** except Vancomycin Resistant *Enterococcus* (VRE) and very rarely reported isolates of Vancomycin Resistant *Staphylococcus aureus* (VRSA)

6. Aminoglycosides

     a. Mechanism: **binds to 30S subunit of bacterial ribosome, blocking protein synthesis initiation and causing misreading of the mRNA code**

     b. Resistance: several major mechanisms described

       1) Altered uptake of the drug

2) Bacterial enzymes stick acetyl groups on aminoglycosides, modifying the drugs' structures, thereby inactivating them
3) Mutations in bacterial ribosomes, blocking the drugs' ability to bind to their targets
4) Anaerobes are intrinsically resistant, as aminoglycosides require an oxidative environment to be transported into the cell

c. Toxicities: **renal tubular damage** and **ototoxicity** are the most prominent toxicities

d. Cidal/Static: cidal

e. Coverage: streptomycin is rarely used, gentamicin is most commonly used, **covers virtually all gram negatives, including nosocomials** like *Pseudomonas*, also **acts synergistically with cell-wall inhibitors** (e.g., penicillins) against gram positives (the cell-wall inhibitors open pores in the cell wall, allowing the bulky aminoglycoside to pass into the cell)

7. Tetracyclines
   a. Mechanism: **binds to 30S subunit of bacterial ribosome, blocking the acceptor site for the incoming aminoacyl-tRNA**, thereby inhibiting protein synthesis
   b. Resistance: due to decreased uptake or actual efflux of the drug from the bacteria mediated by a pump protein
   c. Toxicities: discoloration of teeth in children
   d. Cidal/Static: static
   e. Coverage: doxycycline is by far the most commonly used, **excellent coverage for atypical, intracellular organisms**

8. Chloramphenicol
   a. Mechanism: **binds to the 50S subunit of bacterial ribosome, blocking the action of peptidyltransferase** which inhibits formation of the peptide bond
   b. Resistance: most common mechanism is acetylation of the drug, thereby inactivating it, can also be due to decreased drug uptake
   c. Toxicities:
      1) Dose-dependent aplastic anemia, reversible with cessation of the drug
      2) **Idiosyncratic aplastic anemia, not reversible after drug cessation** and not related to total dose of drug given, **interestingly it has virtually exclusively been reported after oral administration of the drug**, almost never after intravenous administration
      3) **Gray-baby syndrome is due to uncoupling of oxidative phosphorylation** in the myocardium in infants, causing cyanosis and shock

    d. Cidal/Static: static

    e. Coverage: only one drug in the class, very broad spectrum activity, including gram positives, many community-acquired gram negative rods, atypical/intracellular organisms, and many anaerobes, but not considered 1st line for any infections in the developed world

9. Macrolides

    a. Mechanism: **binds to 50S subunit of bacterial ribosome and blocks translocation of amino acids,** interfering with protein synthesis

    b. Resistance: due to decreased cell uptake, enzymatic inactivation of the drugs, or mutations affecting the drugs' binding site on the ribosome

    c. Toxicities: **GI upset with nausea and vomiting is very common with erythromycin,** drug interactions with agents metabolized by cytochrome P450 (such as antihistamines) **causes QT prolongation which can lead to Torsades de Pointes**

    d. Cidal/Static: static

    e. Coverage:

        1) 1st generation: erythromycin is the old stand-by, covers *Streptococcus spp.* and atypicals but has no gram negative coverage, and is still used by some for community acquired pneumonia because it covers many *Streptococcus pneumonia* strains as well as atypicals such as *Mycoplasma* and *Legionella*, **erythromycin is also a reasonable choice to treat penicillin-sensitive infections in penicillin-allergic patients**

        2) 2nd generation: clarithromycin and azithromycin are much better tolerated (less GI adverse effects), have **excellent *Streptococcus* and atypical coverage,** but still minimal gram negative coverage, and are considered first line for outpatient community acquired pneumonia (superior *Streptococcus pneumonia* and atypical coverage, including for *Legionella*), *H. pylori* infection, and *Mycobacterium avium intracellulare*

10. Lincosamide

    a. Mechanism: **binds to 50S subunit of bacterial ribosome and blocks formation of peptide bond**

    b. Resistance: due to mutations altering the drug's binding site on the bacterial ribosomes

    c. Toxicities: **major risk is the triggering of *Clostridium difficile* infection** by wiping out the enteric flora, occurring in up to 10% of patients

    d. Cidal/Static: cidal for gram positive cocci, static for anaerobes

    e. Coverage: clindamycin is the major drug in the class, **first line for anaerobic infections in the lung or oropharynx,** good 2nd line agent for bowel anaerobes (behind metronidazole), also quite good activity against both *Streptococcus* and *Staphylococcus spp.*, making it useful for cellulitis (2nd line behind cephalosporins)

11. Streptogramins
    a. Mechanism: **bind to the 50S subunit of bacterial ribosomes,** inhibiting protein synthesis
    b. Resistance: gram negatives and *Enterococcus faecalis* intrinsically resistant
    c. Toxicities: severe thrombophlebitis, requires central venous access
    d. Cidal/Static: static
    e. Coverage: quinupristin/dalfopristin (Synercid) is the only drug used in this class, **covers most gram positives, including VRE** (but not *E. faecalis*, fortunately most VRE is *E. faecium*), **and MRSA**

12. Oxazolidinone
    a. Mechanism: **binds to the 50S subunit of bacterial ribosomes,** inhibiting protein synthesis by a unique mechanism, that is it **prevents union of the 50S and 30S subunits into the 70S pre-initiation complex,** thereby stopping protein synthesis before it ever begins
    b. Resistance: has been described, but rare
    c. Toxicities: anemia and thrombocytopenia
    d. Cidal/Static: static
    e. Coverage: linezolid is the only drug in this class, approved by the FDA in 2000, **covers essentially all gram positive organisms, including VRE and MRSA**

13. Fluoroquinolones
    a. Mechanism: **blocks activity of DNA gyrase,** which unwinds bacterial DNA during genomic replication
    b. Resistance: due to mutations in DNA gyrase, making it resistant to the drugs' activity
    c. Toxicities: may cause bone or joint disease in children (only convincingly demonstrated in experimental animals), and tendon rupture in adults
    d. Cidal/Static: cidal
    e. Coverage:
        1) **Ciprofloxacin has the best gram negative activity in the class,** best *Pseudomonas* coverage at expense of minimal gram positive coverage, has excellent atypical coverage— excellent drug for kidney (e.g., pyelonephritis), GU (e.g., prostatitis), bowel (e.g., gastroenteritis), & bone (e.g., osteomyelitis)

    2) **Levofloxacin/ofloxacin cover** *Streptococcus* well but not *Staphylococcus*, cover gram negatives but not as well as cipro, and have **excellent atypical coverage**, useful for same infxns as cipro, but also pneumonia

    3) Moxifloxacin/gatifloxacin have extended *Strep* and *Staph* coverage

14. Bactrim (trimethoprim/sulfamethoxazole)
   a. Mechanism: the **trimethoprim blocks dihydrofolate reductase**, inhibiting generation of folate, while **sulfamethoxazole** acts earlier in the folate pathway by acting as a **structural analogue for para-aminobenzoic acid** (PABA), a folate precursor
   b. Resistance: mutations in the folate synthetic pathway and in the enzyme targets
   c. Toxicities: allergic reactions common, ranging from rash to anaphylaxis, rarely folate deficiency may result after prolonged drug intake causing megaloblastic bone marrow suppression
   d. Cidal/Static: cidal
   e. Coverage: Bactrim is a synergistic combination of its two components, good coverage for *Streptococcus* and *Staphylococcus*, good coverage for community acquired gram negative rods (but not nosocomial), **its concentration in the kidney, urine, and prostate make it ideal for uncomplicated UTIs, kidney infections, and GU infections**, and it can be used for community acquired pneumonia, it is also highly active against *Pneumocystic carinii* and *Toxoplasma*, and is used both therapeutically and prophylactically against these organisms

15. Metronidazole
   a. Mechanism: exact target unclear, but it **poisons anaerobic metabolism**
   b. Resistance: unusual, may be due to slow drug uptake
   c. Toxicities: minimal
   d. Cidal/Static: cidal
   e. Coverage: only the one drug in the class, **by far the most effective agent for all bowel anaerobes**, should be used for all biliary, hepatic, and bowel infections and all abscesses in the body, **first line for amebic abscesses**

16. Rifamycins
   a. Mechanism: **inhibit RNA polymerase**
   b. Resistance: **resistance very commonly develops during monotherapy**, requiring that rifamycins always be given in combination with a 2nd agent, mechanism is mutation of bacterial RNA polymerase
   c. Toxicities: turns body secretions red

    d. Cidal/Static: cidal

    e. Coverage: broad spectrum activity when combined with a second agent, 1st line as part of combination chemotherapy for TB, useful as combination therapy for endocarditis or osteomyelitis due to **excellent tissue penetration,** used for close-contact prophylaxis in meningitis due to good salivary penetration, rifampin and rifabutin have similar activities

17. Isoniazid

    a. Mechanism: somehow **inhibits mycolic acid synthesis**

    b. Resistance: develops spontaneously in bacterial chromosomes at a certain set rate, so resistance develops during monotherapy if the organism burden in the patient is high enough to make it statistically possible

    c. Toxicities: **risk of fulminant hepatic toxicity, also commonly depletes vitamin B$_6$**

    d. Cidal/Static: cidal

    e. Coverage: the only drug in the class, extremely effective for TB, also effective against other mycobacteria

B. Fungal Agents

1. Polyenes

    a. Mechanism: **binds to ergosterol in the fungal cell membrane,** punching holes in the membrane

    b. Resistance: rare

    c. Toxicities: extremely toxic agents, very poorly tolerated by patients due to **severe rigors and malaise, invariably causes dose-dependent renal insufficiency, renal tubular acidosis with potassium and magnesium wasting, and bone marrow suppression**

    d. Cidal/Static: cidal

    e. Coverage: nystatin is only used orally and is not absorbed, so it is useful for oropharyngeal or esophageal thrush, while **amphotericin is the mainstay of severe, invasive fungal infections, and should be used for all fungal infections in unstable or neutropenic patients,** liposomal formulations are now available which are less toxic, allowing increasing doses to be administered

2. Azoles

    a. Mechanism: **inhibits ergosterol synthesis by disrupting the cytochrome P450 pathway**

    b. Resistance: some species are intrinsically resistant due to altered P450 enzymes (e.g., *Candida krusei*), resistance is an as-of-yet uncommon but definitely increasing problem

TABLE 6.1	Summary of Antibacterial Antibiotics			
CLASS (EXAMPLE)	**TARGET**	**PROCESS INHIBITED**	**TOXICITY**	**KEY COVERAGE**
Penicillin (PCN)	Transpeptidase	Cell wall synthesis	Allergic	*Strep*, oral anaerobes
Aminopenicillin (ampicillin)	Transpeptidase	Cell wall synthesis	Allergic	*Enterococcus, Listeria*
β-lactamase inhibitor + amp (amp/sulbactam)	Transpeptidase	Cell wall synthesis	Allergic	GPC, GNR, anaerobes but not nosocomials
Penicillinase-resistant PCN (oxacillin)	Transpeptidase	Cell wall synthesis	Allergic	*Staphylococcus* only
Ureidopenicillin (piperacillin)	Transpeptidase	Cell wall synthesis	Allergic	GPC, GNR, anaerobes, & nosocomials
1° Cephalosporin (cefazolin)	Transpeptidase	Cell wall synthesis	Allergic	*Staph/Strep*, some GNR
2° Cephalosporin (cefuroxime)	Transpeptidase	Cell wall synthesis	Allergic	Better *Strep*, better GNR, worse *Staph*
3° Cephalosporin (ceftriazone/ ceftazidime)	Transpeptidase	Cell wall synthesis	Allergic	*Strep* & GNR, nosocomial (ceftazidime)
Carbapenem (imipenem)	Transpeptidase	Cell wall synthesis	Seizure	Broad coverage including nosocomials
Monobactam (aztreonam)	Transpeptidase	Cell wall synthesis	Minimal	GNR including nosocomials
Glycopeptides (vancomycin)	D-alanine-D-alanine	Cell wall synthesis	Allergic	All GPC
Aminoglycoside (gentamicin)	30S ribosome	Protein synthesis	Renal and ototoxic	GNR including nosocomials
Tetracyclines (doxycycline)	50S ribosome	Protein synthesis	Bone/teeth coloration	Atypicals
Chloramphenicol	50S ribosome	Protein synthesis	Bone marrow	Broad but not nosocomials
Macrolide (erythromycin)	50S ribosome	Protein synthesis	GI upset	*Strep* and atypicals

TABLE 6.1	*Continued*			
CLASS (EXAMPLE)	**TARGET**	**PROCESS INHIBITED**	**TOXICITY**	**KEY COVERAGE**
Lincosamide (clindamycin)	50S ribosome	Protein synthesis	*C. difficile*	GPC, for excellent anaerobes
Streptogramin (Synercid)	50S ribosome	Protein synthesis	Thrombophlebitis	VRE and MRSA
Oxazolidinone (linezolid)	50S ribosome	Protein synthesis	Anemia	All GPC
Fluoroquinolones (ciprofloxacin)	DNA gyrase	DNA replication	Bone/joint damage	*Strep*, GNR, nosocomials, atypicals
Bactrim	PABA/ dihydrofolate reductase	Folate synthesis	Allergic	GPC, GNR, protozoa
Metronidazole	Unclear	Anaerobic metabolism	Minimal	1st line anaerobes
Rifamycins (rifampin)	RNA polymerase	RNA transcription	Red urine & tears	GPC, GNR, atypicals
Isoniazid	Unclear	Mycolic acid synthesis	Hepatic, deplete B6	*Mycobacteria*

c. Toxicities: GI intolerance, cholestasis, hepatitis are the most common
d. Cidal/Static: static
e. Coverage: although miconazole and clotrimazole are used topically, fluconazole and itraconazole are really the only two azoles still used for invasive disease, **fluconazole has excellent *Candida*, *Cryptococcus*, and *Coccidioides* coverage (that is, it hits yeast very well), but it doesn't cover molds at all, whereas itraconazole has reasonable *Aspergillus* coverage but is less well tolerated than fluconazole,** so use fluconazole for all yeast infections and itraconazole for *Aspergillus*

VII. OVERVIEW OF CLASS A BIOTERRORISM PATHOGENS

TABLE 7.1	Overview of Class A Bioterrorism Pathogens		
PATHOGEN	**KEY BUZZWORDS**	**Dx**	**Tx**
B. anthracis	• Rapidly progressive pneumonia with sepsis or painless necrotic eschar on skin with lymphadenopathy • Widened mediastinum on CXR • Postal worker or association with opening of mail	Gram stain → GPR, culture grows the organism	Fluoroquinolone ± doxycycline empirically until sensitivities back—strongly consider aminoglycoside as well
Y. pestis	• Rapidly progressive pneumonia with sepsis or bubos in axilla/groin • Community acquired gram negative rods in sputum or in blood cultures	Gram stain → GNR, culture grows the organism	Fluoroquinolone ± doxycycline—consider aminoglycoside as well
F. tularensis	• Progressive flu-like illness, followed by sepsis, possibly with necrotic eschar(s) on skin	Gram stain → gram negative coccobacilli	Aminoglycoside, fluoroquinolones & doxycycline have activity
C. botulinum	• Cranial neuropathies, drooling, diplopia, symmetric descending weakness	Contact public health	Supportive care, anti-toxin
Smallpox (Variola)	• Flu-like illness with papulo-pustular rash starting on face and extremities and uniformly progresses so all lesions at same stage	Contact public health	Supportive, VIG for progressive vaccinia, severe generalized vaccinia
Ebola/ Marburg	• Petechiae, hemorrhage, thrombocytopenia, hypotension	Contact public health	Supportive

MICROBIOLOGY REVIEW

QUESTIONS

1. A 50-year-old man complains for several days of a cough productive of greenish sputum. He has a fever of 101°F, an infiltrate on CXR, and a positive sputum culture. What laboratory test pattern is the most likely for the organism growing from his sputum?
    a) GPC in clusters, coagulase positive
    b) GPC in chains, β-hemolytic
    c) GPC in pairs, quellung positive
    d) GPC in chains, CAMP factor positive
    e) GPC in pairs, resistant to hypertonic saline

2. Gram stain of a clinical specimen reveals gram positive cocci in pairs and chains. Laboratory testing reveals resistance to bile, hydrolysis of esculin, and resistance to hypertonic saline. Susceptibility testing reveals resistance to penicillin and vancomycin. What antibiotic would you recommend for coverage?
    a) Ampicillin
    b) Ampicillin + sulbactam
    c) Gentamicin
    d) Imepenem
    e) Linezolid

3. Match the following gastrointestinal toxidromes with their causative organism:

1) *E. coli* O157:H7	a) Reheated fried rice
2) *S. aureus*	b) Onset of sx at 6 hr after consumption
3) *Bacillus cereus*	c) Onset 16 hr after eating reheated food
4) *Vibrio cholera*	d) ADP-ribosylation of G-protein in intestinal cells
5) *C. perfringens*	e) Hemolytic-uremic syndrome

4. A 60-year-old alcoholic male is brought into the emergency room after being found down on the street. The patient is confused but not tremulous. His alcohol level is zero. He is febrile and tachycardic, and has meningismus on exam. His lumbar puncture shows a thousand white cells, consistent with meningitis. What antibiotics should be started for this patient and why?

   a) Ceftriaxone to cover for *Streptococcus pneumonia, Hemophilus,* and *Neisseria meningitidis*

   b) Ceftazadime to cover for *Pseudomonas*

   c) Ceftriaxone and gentamicin to cover for *S. pneumonia, Hemophilus, Neisseria,* and *Listeria*

   d) Ampicillin and ceftriaxone to cover for *S. pneumonia, Hemophilus, Neisseria,* and *Listeria*

   e) Ceftriaxone to cover *S. pneumonia, Hemophilus,* and *Neisseria,* and gentamicin for synergistic coverage for *Streptococcus agalactiae*

5. Match the following immunodeficiencies with the organisms to which they impart susceptibility (each immunodeficiency can only be used once!):

1) Splenectomy	a) BK Polyomavirus
2) CD4 count <200	b) *Aspergillus* dissemination
3) Neutropenia	c) *Neisseria meningitidis*
4) C6 deficiency	d) *Streptococcus pneumonia*
5) Renal transplant	e) *Pneumocystis jiruveci*

6. The following are defining characteristics of Enterobacteriaceae **except:**

   a) Facultative anaerobes

   b) Ferment lactose

   c) Oxidase negative

   d) Ferment glucose

   e) Reduce nitrates to nitrites

7. Match the following diseases to their most common etiological agent (each bacteria can be used once, more than once or not at all):

1) Meningitis in adults	a) *E. coli*
2) Community acquired pneumonia	b) *Campylobacter*
3) Urinary tract infection	c) *Streptococcus pneumonia*
4) Gastroenteritis in the U.S.	d) *Streptococcus agalactiae*
5) Meningitis in neonates	e) *Staphylococcus aureus*

8. Match the following organisms with special requirements for culture:
   1) *Hemophilus influenza*   a) Iron and cysteine supplements
   2) *Corynebacterium*   b) Lowenstein–Jensen medium
   3) *Neisseria gonorrhoeae*   c) Tellurite agar
   4) *Legionella*   d) Thayer–Martin agar
   5) TB   e) Factor V & Factor X

9. Match the following causes of community acquired pneumonia with its special characteristics:
   1) *S. aureus*   a) Diarrhea, hyponatremia, very high LDH
   2) *Acinetobacter*   b) Lung abscesses following aspiration pneumonia
   3) *Klebsiella*   c) Follows antecedent influenza
   3) *Klebsiella*   d) Nosocomial pneumonia in ICU patients on ventilators
   4) *Legionella*   e) "Currant-jelly" hemoptysis, often in diabetics or alcoholics
   5) *Bacteroides*

10. Match the following zoonotic organisms with their risks for transmission?
    1) *Brucella*   a) Dog bite
    2) *Francisella*   b) Milk and farm animals
    3) *Pasteurella*   c) Flea
    4) *Yersinia pestis*   d) Tick

11. Match the following patients with the appropriate PPD diameter for treating with isoniazid (letters can be used more than once):
    1) A 30-year-old homeless man   a) 5 mm
    2) A 25-year-old healthy male   b) 10 mm
    3) A 40-year-old healthy male with no risks   c) 15 mm
    4) A 60-year-old pt with old dz on CXR   d) No tx
    5) A 45-year-old male with AIDS

12. Which of the following spirochetes does **not** cause significant CNS disease?
    a) *Treponema pallidum*
    b) *Borrelia burgdorferi*
    c) *Borrelia recurrentis*
    d) *Leptospira*

13. Which of the following is not a risk factor for invasive candidiasis?
    a) AIDS
    b) Neutropenia
    c) Central venous catheters
    d) Parenteral nutrition
    e) Laparotomy

14. Match the following risk factors with the appropriate fungus:

    1) Pigeon droppings   a) *Histoplasma*
    2) Spelunking   b) *Sporothrix*
    3) Antibiotics   c) *Rhizopus*
    4) Serum pH 7.20   d) *Candida*
    5) Rose bushes   e) *Cryptococcus*

15. Which of the following protozoa commonly causes abscesses?
    a) *Cryptosporidium*
    b) *Entamoeba*
    c) *Giardia*
    d) *Trichomonas*

16. Match the following invasive protozoa with their appropriate vectors:

    1) *Leishmania*   a) Reduviid bug
    2) *Plasmodium*   b) Sandfly
    3) *Trypanosoma cruzi*   c) Tsetse fly
    4) *Trypanosoma gambiense*   d) *Anopheles* mosquito

17. Which of the following statements regarding *Plasmodium* infections is **not** true?
    a) *P. falciparum* malaria is phenotypically the most severe
    b) Tertian fevers occur every 48 hr
    c) Quartan fever can be treated with chloroquine alone
    d) Tertian fever can be treated with primaquine alone
    e) Resistance to quinines is becoming a worldwide problem

18. Match the following helminths to the exposures most likely to result in their infection (exposures may be used more than once):

    1) *Diphyllobothrium*   a) Raw crab meat
    2) *Echinococcus*   b) Raw pork
    3) *Taenia saginata*   c) Raw fish
    4) *Taenia solium*   d) Dogs and sheep
    5) *Clonorchis sinensis*   e) Raw beef
    6) *Paragonimus westermani*
    7) *Trichinella spiralis*

19. Which of the following statements is **false**?
    a) Hookworms are the leading cause of iron deficiency anemia worldwide
    b) *Ascaris* is the most common helminthic infection worldwide
    c) *Enterobius* is the most common helminthic infection in the U.S.
    d) *Trichiuris* causes rectal prolapse
    e) Prominent eosinophilia occurs in all parasitic infections

20. Match the following viruses to the diseases they cause:
    1) Adenovirus   a) Roseola infantum
    2) JC Polyomavirus   b) Heterophile negative mononucleosis
    3) Parvovirus B19   c) Breakbone fever
    4) Cytomegalovirus   d) Kaposi's sarcoma
    5) HHV 6   e) Herpangina
    6) HHV 8   f) Progressive multifocal leukoencephalopathy
    7) Coxsackievirus   g) Tropical spastic paraparesis
    8) Dengue Virus   h) 5th disease, erythema infectiosum
    9) HTLV   i) Pharyngoconjunctival fever

21. Which of the following statements regarding Hepatitis B Virus is **false**?
    a) Hepatitis B Virus e antigen titers correlate with infectivity of the patient
    b) The most common mode of transmission worldwide is vertical
    c) The "window period" is when the Hepatitis B Virus surface antigen is negative but the surface antibody test is positive
    d) Hepatitis B Virus has a reverse transcriptase
    e) Whereas Hepatitis B Surface Antibody correlates with immunity to infection the Hepatitis B Core Antibody is not protective

22. Match the following antibiotics with the biochemical step they inhibit:
    1) Penicillin   a) Amino acid translocation
    2) Gentamicin   b) Dihydrofolate reductase
    3) Doxycycline   c) Mycolic acid synthesis
    4) Chloramphenicol   d) Peptidyltransferase
    5) Erythromycin   e) Formation of 70S
    6) Clindamycin   f) RNA polymerase
    7) Linezolid   g) Proper reading of mRNA codons
    8) Ciprofloxacin   h) Transpeptidase
    9) Bactrim   i) Aminoacyl-tRNA binding
    10) Rifampin   j) Peptide bond formation
    11) Isoniazid   k) DNA gyrase

Questions 23–25 refer to a 23-year-old registered nurse who arrives in your outpatient clinic at the completion of her night shift at the local community hospital. She tells you that she has a history of intermittent nasal pain, and intermittent nasal erythema, which occasionally spreads to her cheeks. She is usually able to get one of the doctors at the hospital to give her some oral antibiotics but this time they haven't worked to get rid of the infection. Also, she now complains of headache, fever, and severe nasal pain, swelling and redness. Pt has no significant past medical history or any known drug allergies.

Physical exam: She is an alert, otherwise healthy appearing female, VS-101.8, 106, 18, 130/86. She has erythema and swelling of her nose, and purulence noted within the nasal vestibule. No nuchal rigidity, no photophobia, and her WBC count is moderately elevated.

23. What organism is most likely causing this patient's cellulitis?
    a) Coccobacillus with bipolar staining
    b) Gram negative rods shaped like a comma
    c) Gram positive rods with square ends in a chain
    d) Gram positive cocci in clusters

24. What is the most likely organism involved in this patient's infection?
    a) *Pseudomonas*
    b) *E. coli*
    c) Resistant *S. aureus*
    d) Resistant *Enterococcus spp.*

25. You have decided to admit this patient to the hospital for inpatient intravenous antibiotic therapy. You obtain cultures of the purulent drainage in her nose. You decide to empirically treat her infection until her cultures return with which of the following antibiotics?
    a) Ceftriaxone
    b) Cefazolin
    c) Vancomycin
    d) Metronidazole
    e) Ciprofloxacin

ANSWERS

1. **c)** *Streptococcus pneumonia* is the most common cause of community acquired pneumonia. *S. pneumonia* is gram positive and often described as "*diplococcus*," meaning pairs of cocci, although it can also grow in chains (so "pairs and chains" is often seen). *S. pneumonia* is α-hemolytic, not β-hemolytic, and it has a prominent polysaccharide capsule which causes the quellung test to be positive. GPC in clusters refers to *Staphylococcus*, and the positive coagulase test would identify *S. aureus*. β-hemolytic GPC in chains could be any of the "grouped" *Streptococci* (e.g., Group A, Group B, etc.). CAMP factor identifies Group B Strep, and GPC resistant to hypertonic saline identifies *Enterococcus*.

2. **e)** Gram positive cocci in pairs and chains resistant to bile that hydrolyzes esculin could be either *Streptococcus bovis* or *Enterococcus*. The resistance to hypertonic saline identifies the organism as *Enterococcus*, and the resistance to vancomycin identifies vancomycin resistant *Enterococcus* (VRE). As the VRE is also resistant to penicillin (which is often the case), linezolid (or quinupristin/dalfopristin, which wasn't one of the choices) must be used.

3. **1-e, 2-b, 3-a, 4-d, 5-c.** *S. aureus* exotoxin causes nausea, vomiting, and diarrhea within 8 hr of consumption of contaminated food. *Bacillus cereus* also causes rapid onset of symptoms, typically within 4 hr of consumption, although a longer incubation can also be seen. The classic buzz word for *B. cereus* gastroenteritis is the reheating of fried rice, which causes bacterial endospores to activate. In contrast *Clostridium perfringens* gastroenteritis typically occurs 8–16 hr after food consumption. *E. coli* O157:H7 secretes a Shiga-like toxin which can cause a severe inflammatory gastroenteritis, and in children can cause the hemolytic-uremic syndrome. *Vibrio cholera* toxin ADP-ribosylates a G-protein linked to an ion channel, allowing constant secretion of fluid and salt into the gut. This results in a secretory diarrhea.

4. **d)** The key to this question is the presence of meningitis in a compromised host. Specifically, alcoholism is associated with an increased susceptibility to *Listeria* meningitis (as is, for example, diabetes or any other chronic, debilitating illness). Ceftriaxone is empiric therapy of choice for all community acquired meningitis, but it does not cover *Listeria*. In general aminopenicillins, such as ampicillin, are the best coverage for *Listeria*, and must be added in this case.

5. **1-d, 2-e, 3-b, 4-c, 5-a.** Splenectomy results in relative suppression of antibody responses to blood-born infections. For microbes with anti-phagocytic polysaccharide capsules antibody production is key to host protection, as the antibody opsonizes the otherwise non-phagocytosable organism. Thus, splenectomy makes hosts susceptible to bacteremia caused by microbes with polysaccharide capsules, of

which *S. pneumonia* is the most common example. AIDS patients with CD4 counts less than 200 are at markedly increased risk for developing *Pneumocystis* pneumonia. Neutropenia is the major risk factor for developing disseminated fungal infections, particularly for *Aspergillus* and *Candida*, but also for *Mucor* and others. Deficiencies in the late components of the complement cascade (C5–C9), impart susceptibility to *Neisseria* infections. Renal transplant patients can develop nephritis from the BK Polyomavirus.

6.   **b)** Enterobacteriaceae are all facultative anaerobes that ferment glucose, reduce nitrates to nitrites, and are oxidase negative. Only some (e.g., *E. coli*, *Enterobacter*, and *Klebsiella*) ferment lactose.

7.   **1-c, 2-c, 3-a, 4-b, 5-d.** *Streptococcus pneumonia* is the most common cause of community acquired pneumonia and meningitis in adults in the U.S. *Campylobacter* is the most common cause of invasive gastroenteritis in the U.S., while *E. coli* is the most common cause of urinary tract infections. Group B strep is the number one cause of meningitis in neonates.

8.   **1-e, 2-c, 3-d, 4-a, 5-b.**

9.   **1-c, 2-d, 3-e, 4-a, 5-b.** *S. aureus* is a very uncommon cause of community acquired pneumonia. It occurs in two major settings: as a post-viral bacterial process or due to seeding of the lungs caused by *Staphylococcal* bacteremia. *Acinetobacter* is only seen in the nosocomial setting, typically in patients on ventilators. *Klebsiella* causes a necrotic lung process leading to prominent hemoptysis with thick, bloody mucous, described as "currant jelly." *Legionella* causes severe pneumonia associated with diarrhea, hyponatremia, and very high LDH. *Bacteroides* is an obligate anaerobe. The only time it can exist in the lung is in a polymicrobial abscess where the oxygen is utilized by facultative anaerobes.

10.   **1-b, 2-d, 3-a, 4-c.** *Pasteurella* is typically transmitted from an animal bite, usually dog or cat. *Yersinia* is transmitted by fleas, which have fed on rodents, while *Francisella* is spread by ticks having fed on rabbits or other mammals. *Brucella* is transmitted during contact with farm animals.

11.   **1-b, 2-c, 3-c, 4-a, 5-a.** Patients with "high risk" for TB, including those with HIV, those in contact with people who have active disease, those with debilitating illnesses (such as renal failure or cancer), and those with evidence of old TB on CXR, should receive INH therapy if their PPDs are ≥5 mm. People with risk factors such as homelessness, imprisonment, immigration from high-risk areas (such as Latin America and Asia), and employment in health care should be treated if their PPDs are ≥10 mm. Healthy adults with no risk factors should be treated if they have PPDs ≥15 mm. In the past, these latter patients would not have received INH if they were over 35 yrs old.

However, the updated guidelines from 2000 no longer take age into account for the decision to give INH. If you place a PPD and it is positive, the patient should be treated. On the other hand, the guidelines recommend not placing PPDs on elderly people without TB risks.

12. **c)** Syphilis (*T. pallidum*), Lyme disease (*B. burgdorferi*), and Weil's disease (*Leptospira*) all cause prominent aseptic meningitis. *B. recurrentis* causes undulating fevers with lymphadenopathy.

13. **a)** For unclear reasons, AIDS patients get oral-mucosal candidiasis, but not invasive disease. Each of the other factors, along with broad spectrum antibiotics, are risks for invasive candidiasis. Any GI surgery, such as laparotomy, is a significant risk.

14. **1-e, 2-a, 3-d, 4-c, 5-b.** Although it is not clear if this is of any clinical significance, *Cryptococcus* is found at high levels in pigeon droppings, and there is a theoretical risk of contracting the disease from people with prolonged contact to pigeon droppings. Spelunking, or cave exploration, is a classic risk factor for *Histoplasma*, which is found at high concentrations in bat droppings. Administration of broad-spectrum antibiotics is a risk factor for invasive candidiasis. Metabolic acidosis, probably due to inhibition of host phagocytes, is the major risk factor for development of mucormycosis, an infection caused by *Mucor* or *Rhizopus*. Finally, *Sporothrix* is inoculated into the body after a skin break caused by thorns. The classic boards question is a gardener who develops fevers and ascending lymphadenopathy in one arm.

15. **b)** *Entamoeba* is the cause of amoebic liver abscess.

16. **1-b, 2-d, 3-a, 4-c.**

17. **d)** Tertian fevers occur on every 3rd day, or every 48 hr, while quartan fevers occur on every 4th day, or every 72 hr. The organisms which cause tertian fever, *P. vivax* and *P. ovale*, both reside in the liver. Chloroquine treats the blood-born merozoites, but does not penetrate into the dormant liver forms, allowing recrudescence to occur. Chloroquine plus primaquine should be used in such patients. Conversely, *P. malaria* causes quartan fevers and has no liver phase. It can be treated successfully with chloroquine alone. *P. falciparum* does cause the most severe malaria, due to higher organism burdon and the risk of microcapillary thrombosis in the brain. Resistance to quinine derivatives is becoming a global problem.

18. **1-c, 2-d, 3-e, 4-b, 5-c, 6-a, 7-b.** *Diphyllobothrium* and *Clonorchis* are transmitted via ingestion of undercooked fish. *Echinococcus* can be transmitted from ingestion of eggs in dog feces or via consumption of undercooked sheep meat. Raw pork can transmit either *Taenia solium* or *Trichinella*, while raw beef can transmit *Taenia saginata* and raw crab meat can transmit *Paragonimus*.

19. **e)** Eosinophilia only occurs during infections caused by parasites that invade tissues. Tapeworms, for example, which only reside in the intestinal lumen, do not cause eosinophilia.

20. **1-i, 2-f, 3-h, 4-b, 5-a, 6-d, 7-e, 8-c, 9-g.**

21. **c)** The window period occurs when the immune system begins to clear viral antigens from the serum, but the antibody response has not yet achieved a titer which is detectable by lab assays. The immunodominant antigen of HBV is the surface antigen. Thus the window period is when the surface antigen has been cleared and thus is negative, but the titer of the surface antibody is not yet high enough to be detectable. Often during this period the antibody to the HBV core antigen is positive, as these antibodies seem to be produced earlier on. Thus the window period is typified by negative surface antigen, and positive core antibody, and negative surface antibody.

22. **1-h, 2-g, 3-i, 4-d, 5-a, 6-j, 7-e, 8-k, 9-b, 10-f, 11-c.**

23. **d)** Gram positive cocci in clusters. Most commonly skin related infections are caused by gram positive cocci. Hospital staff are commonly colonized within their nasal cavities with these infections. The cluster formation on Gram stain is commonly seen in the *Staphylococcus spp.* *Pasteurella multocida* is a common cause of dog or cat bite cellulitis and presents as a small coccobacillus with bipolar staining on Gram stain and is unlikely the cause. Gram negative rods shaped like a comma are commonly found in enteric infections caused by *Vibrio cholera*. *Bacillus anthracis* appears like box cars on Gram stain (GPR with square ends in a chain) is also unlikely to be the cause of this patient's cellulitis.

24. **c)** Resistant *S. aureus* as mentioned earlier is the most likely cause of this patient's nasal cellulitis. Her history of previous relief with oral antibiotics is a hint of infection with a resistant strain of *Staphylococcus*. Although *Pseudomonas*, *Enteroccocus*, and *E.coli* are common nosocomial infections they rarely infect staff unless they are immuno-compromised or have open wounds and poor hand-washing.

25. **c)** Vancomycin. This patient has most likely been treated previously with oral antibiotics that cover normal skin flora (i.e., gram positive cocci). The ongoing infection of her nose despite antibiotics strongly suggests the infecting pathogen may be drug-resistant (i.e., MRSA). Therefore, vancomycin is the preferred antibiotic. If sensitivities return as methicillin sensitive *S. aureus*, the vancomycin can be stopped and a beta lactam can be started.

Immunology

VIII. WHITE BLOOD CELLS (LEUKOCYTES)

A. Myeloid Cells

1. Granulocytes
   a. Neutrophils
      1) Most numerous WBCs (40–70% of total), short-lived (lifespan = 6–12 hrs)
      2) Neutrophil production in the bone marrow is stimulated by **granulocyte-colony stimulating factor** (G–CSF = Neupogen), which is used clinically for neutropenia
      3) Neutrophils contain two types of cytoplasmic granules
         a) Primary granules contain small **cationic proteins called defensins,** which are inherently toxic to microbes, as well as the enzyme **myeloperoxidase**, which kills microbes via generation of hypochlorous acid (i.e., bleach)
         b) Secondary granules contain iron chelators and degradative enzymes
      4) Like all phagocytes, **neutrophils are intrinsically non-specific and without memory,** however like all phagocytes they are capable of **antibody-dependent cell-mediated cytotoxicity (ADCC)**
         a) ADCC is when a phagocyte binds to the Fc (constant) portion of an antibody that is attached by its variable region to a microbe
         b) The antibody thus provides **specificity** to a non-specific leukocyte, enabling it to target lytic enzyme secretions to the bound microbe
      5) Dead neutrophils comprise pus
   b. Eosinophils
      1) **Play a role in parasitic defense,** utilizing IgE-dependent ADCC to secrete special anti-eukaryotic toxins onto parasites
      2) Involved in asthma/allergy via IgE-provided antigen specificity
      3) Differential diagnosis of peripheral eosinophilia (defined as 500 eosinophils/μL): the **NAACP mnemonic**
         a) **N**eoplasm (often leukemia/lymphoma)/Nocardia
         b) **A**llergy/**A**sthma/**A**topy
         c) **A**spergillus infections/Addison's disease
         d) **C**ollagen-Vascular dz/Coccidioides
         e) **P**arasitic infections—note that parasites that cause eosinophilia are almost all multicellular (helminths in particular) that cross tissue planes; intestinal parasites often do not cause eosinophilia, and the only protozoa that typically causes eosinophilia is *Isospora*

    c. Basophils
      1) Rare cells (<1% of total), bind to IgE Fc region
      2) Regulate vascular tone, can affect IgE-mediated Type I Hypersensitivity (see below)
    d. Mast Cells
      1) Tissue cells, not typically found in the blood
      2) A myeloid cell of separate lineage from basophils (contrary to popular opinion, these are not tissue basophils)
      3) **Responsible for IgE-mediated Type I Hypersensitivity**

2. Mononuclear Cells
    a. Monocytes
      1) Comprise 1–10% of WBCs, long-lived cells
      2) Circulate in blood, eventually extravasate into tissues to become macrophages
    b. Macrophages
      1) The terminally differentiated form of monocytes
      2) **These are the most phagocytic cells in the body**
      3) Are massive factories for cytokine production
      4) Destroy senescent RBCs in spleen and other tissues
      5) Act as professional Antigen Presenting Cells (APCs)
        a) **Professional APCs express Class II Major Histocompatibility Complex (MHC)**
        b) Class II MHC molecules allow professional APCs to present antigen to T-helper cells

3. Megakaryocytes
    a. Multinucleated giant cells (**the only polyploid cells in the body**)
    b. Have up to 32 or 64 times the normal cell DNA content
    c. Formed by precursors undergoing repeated DNA replication without cell division
    d. Act as factories which produce platelets by cell membrane budding
    e. Platelets secrete potent antimicrobial peptides similar to defensins

4. Dendritic Cells
    a. Not found in blood at high levels
    b. **The most efficient APCs in the body** (less phagocytic than macrophages but more efficient at antigen presentation due to more efficient co-stimulation of T cells)
    c. Reside in epithelial and lymph tissues most of the time— **Langerhans cells are a special population of dendritic cells found in the skin**

d. Dendritic cells sample their environments by phagocytosing antigen
e. After taking up antigen, dendritic cells migrate via vasculature to the spleen or via lymph channels to lymph nodes, and initiate immune responses by activating T cells

B. Lymphoid Cells

1. B Lymphocytes
   a. **Identifiable by surface expression of antibody, which serves as the B-cell receptor**
      1) **Antibodies are tetramers composed of two identical heavy chain molecules and two identical light chain molecules** (see Figure 8.1)
      2) **Both heavy and light chain molecules have constant regions and variable regions**
         a) Constant regions of heavy chains come in one of five varieties, defining the antibody subtype: IgM, IgD, IgG, IgE, and IgA (Mnemonic: **M**edical **D**octors **G**ive **E**veryone **A**spirin)
         b) Constant regions of light chains come in one of two varieties, defining the light chain subtype: kappa (κ) or lambda (λ)
         c) **Both heavy chain and light chain variable regions are created by genetic recombination events, allowing generation of up to 10^{12} unique sequences** (see Figure 8.2)

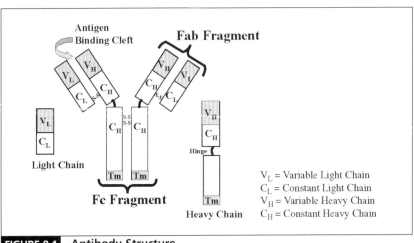

FIGURE 8.1 Antibody Structure

S-S, disulfide bond; Tm, transmembrane region.

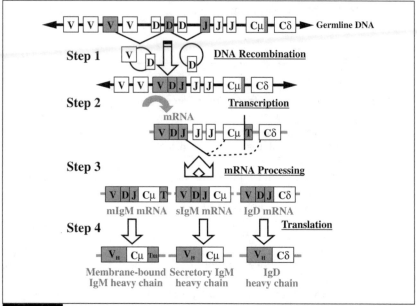

FIGURE 8.2 **Recombination of Antibody Genes**

Antibody diversity is generated by recombination of DNA cassettes to create a variable region for both the light and heavy chains of an antibody (only heavy chain recombination is depicted here). The germline DNA of all cells contains hundreds of Variable (V) and dozens of Diversity (D) and Joining (J) segments in the immunoglobulin loci, each of which can be randomly recombined to become part of a gene coding for antibody. Step 1) The first recombination event fuses a randomly selected D region with a J region, excising from the chromosome all the DNA in between. This is followed by recombination joining a random V segment with the D–J fusion product, again excising intervening DNA from the chromosome. Step 2) mRNA is transcribed from the 5′ leader sequence of the V–D–J segment to the 3′ terminus of the genes coding for the IgM (Cμ) and IgD (Cδ) constant regions. Step 3) Nucleotides intervening between the V–D–J variable region and the IgM and IgD constant region genes are excised from the mRNA, resulting in either mature IgM or IgD mRNA. Due to alternative splicing, naïve B cells co-express IgM and IgD bearing the same variable region on the cell surface. In addition, the 3′ end of the IgM constant region gene (Cμ) contains a second alternative splice site followed by a short transmembrane domain (Tm). If the Tm is not spliced out, the IgM will attach to the cell membrane (mIgM) and serve as a surface receptor. Following B-cell activation, the Tm will be spliced out, allowing the activated B cell to secrete its antibody (sIgM). IgD is not normally secreted. Step 4) Translation of the mature mRNA into its polypeptide product.

TABLE 8.1	Characteristics of IG Subtypes
SUBTYPE	**CHARACTERISTICS**
IgM	• Secreted by newly activated naïve B cells • **Marker of primary exposure to antigen** • **Forms pentamers in serum**, J chain joins the monomers by binding to their constant regions • Fixes complement well
IgD	• Expressed with IgM on the surface of naïve B cells
IgG	• Secreted by differentiated/memory B cells • **Marker of re-exposure to antigen** • Always monomeric in serum • Fixes complement well • **Crosses the placenta**
IgE	• Secreted by differentiated/memory B cells • **Causes allergy/asthma by binding to receptors on mast cells and basophils and inducing degranulation** • **Kills parasites** by inducing eosinophil-mediated ADCC
IgA	• Secreted by **mucosal B cells** • Forms dimers, joined by J chain binding to constant region • Epithelial cells translocate IgA dimers by binding to the J chain, and then exocytose the IgA on the mucosal surface, **resulting in high IgA levels in mucosal secretions**

      d) The heavy and light chain variable regions intertwine, forming a cleft to bind to antigen—**therefore specificity of an antibody for its antigen is determined by the sequences of heavy and light chain variable regions**

   3) The antibody molecule can be divided into domains (see Figure 8.1)

      a) **The Fab domain is the antigen-binding region** formed by the variable regions of heavy and light chains

      b) **The Fc domain is the constant portion of the heavy chain which defines the antibody subtype (e.g., IgM vs. IgG)**

   4) **By alternative splicing of mRNA** transcribed from the recombined antibody gene, **the B cell can either express a membrane bound form of the antibody** (the B-cell receptor) or can remove the membrane binding section of the constant region allowing **secretion of the antibody** (see Figures 8.1 and 8.2)

    5) Allelic exclusion

       a) **Allelic exclusion ensures all the antibody expressed by a given B cell is specific for the same antigen (to a first approximation)**

       b) After recombination successfully generates a functional heavy chain gene, a signal is sent to the cell to stop recombining the other allele, thereby excluding expression of both alleles

       c) Allelic exclusion also functions during recombination of the light chain allele

       d) Therefore all antibodies express only one heavy chain allele and one light chain allele, and thus can make antibodies with only one variable region specificity (to a first approximation)

  b. B cells develop in the bone marrow, then migrate to lymphatic tissues to seek out the antigen for which they are specific

  c. Antigen

    1) Antigen is broadly defined as any molecule to which an immune response can be generated

    2) Practically speaking, most antigens are proteins; however, antibodies can be generated to any chemical, including those not normally found in the body

  d. **Clonal Selection Activation** (see Figure 8.3)

    1) The body contains billions of B cells, each of which produces antibody with a unique antigen-binding specificity

    2) Appropriate antibody responses are generated when antigen binds to, or selects, the few clones of B cells among the billions in the body whose antibody is specific for that antigen

    3) The antigen-specific B cells are then activated (see the following) and given signals to proliferate, resulting in selective expansion of only those clones reactive to the antigen

  e. Two-Signal Lymphocyte Activation

    1) Antigen cross-links antibody in the B cell membrane, resulting in Signal 1, the first of two signals required to activate the B cell

    2) **Despite antigen ligation of surface antibody, B cells cannot be fully activated to make antibody against protein antigens unless T-helper cells are available to provide a second stimulatory signal (Signal 2)**

    3) Signal 2

       a) T-cell second signal is provided by surface binding of CD40-ligand on the T cell to CD40 on the B cell, as well as by T-cell secretion of helper cytokines such as IL-4, IL-10, and IL-13, which enable B-cell proliferation and activation of antibody secretion

B Lymphocytes

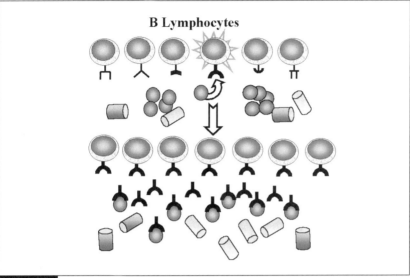

FIGURE 8.3 Clonal Selection Activation of Lymphocytes

Naïve B-cells with diverse antigen-specific receptors circulate through the lymphatics scanning for an activating antigen. Antigens selectively activate B cells whose antibody receptors specifically recognize the antigen. This leads to proliferation and expansion of those particular B-cell clones, which then secrete an excess of antibody to clear the antigen from the host.

  b) The second signal provided by T cells is a safety check to prevent B cells from being activated by host antigens

  c) If a B cell binds to antigen but no T cell has been activated by that same antigen, the B cell undergoes apoptosis

4) **There are two classes of T-cell independent antigens which can stimulate B cell production of antibody without T cell help (e.g., without Signal 2)**

  a) Type 1 T-cell independent antigens

   i) These are all mitogens, which inherently stimulate B-cell proliferation without binding to the B-cell receptor (e.g., without generating Signal 1)

   ii) The most famous Type 1 T-cell independent antigen is gram negative bacterial lipopolysaccharide (endotoxin, a non-secreted substance that is part of the bacterial cell wall that induces massive inflammation), which binds to CD14 and the Toll-4 receptor on the B-cell surface

      iii) **Thus lipopolysaccharide, like all Type 1 T-cell indepen-
dent antigens, bypasses both Signal 1 and Signal 2**
and generates a completely different activating signal
(lipopolysaccharide binding to CD14 and Toll-4)

   b) Type 2 T-cell independent antigens

      i)   Large polysaccharide molecules with multiple repeating
sequences, such as those found in bacterial cell walls,
can cross-link B-cell receptors so effectively that T-cell
help is not needed for activation

      ii) **Thus, unlike Type I T-cell independent antigen, Type II
T-cell independent antigens do bind to the B-cell
receptor to generate Signal 1, and bypass Signal 2 by
generating such a powerful Signal 1 that Signal 2 is
simply irrelevant**

      iii) Examples of T-cell independent antigens are *Hemophilus
influenza* and *Streptococus pneumonia* capsular
polysaccharide—vaccines based on these polysaccha-
rides had to be chemically linked to protein carrier
molecules to allow T-cell activation significant long-
term vaccine-mediated protection

f. B cells activated in the presence of T-helper cells differentiate
into plasma cells that can produce antibodies—**these are the
primary effectors of humoral immunity**

g. **Differentiation into plasma cells occurs in the germinal centers
of lymph nodes**

h. During plasma cell differentiation, two processes occur that
change the nature of the secreted antibodies

   1) **Class switching**

     a) Deletion of intervening DNA allows an antibody to switch
from IgM to IgG subtype (see Figure 8.4)

     b) Additional class switching allows change from IgG to IgE to
IgA

     c) IgM is thus a marker for naïve and newly activated B cells,
whereas IgG is a marker of a mature plasma cell or a
memory B cell

     d) **Class switching cannot occur without T cell help** (thus T-cell
independent antigens can only stimulate IgM antibodies,
not IgG)

   2) **Affinity maturation**

     a) During the differentiation of B cells to plasma cells, the
germ line DNA coding for the antibody is susceptible to a
million-fold increase in its mutation rate

     b) As the maturing plasma cells continue to divide, this
increased mutation rate generates individual clones with
slightly different germ line DNA, coding for antibodies of
slightly different specificity

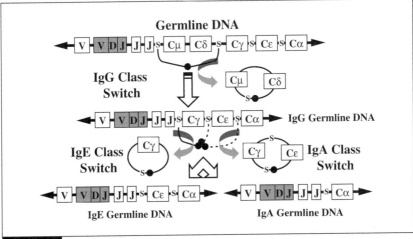

Germline DNA

FIGURE 8.4 | **Ig Class Switching**

Class switching is the swap of the same variable region onto a different heavy chain constant region, e.g., switching IgM to variable IgG during an immune response. B cells undergo this process in the germinal centers of lymph nodes. Class switching occurs via intrachromosomal recombination targeted to special switch sites (S) 5' to each constant region gene. All IgMs must class-switch to IgG before proceeding to IgE or IgA. During this initial class switch, DNA coding for the constant region of IgM and IgD (Cμ and Cδ) are excised from the chromosome. Subsequent class switching from IgG can either proceed to IgE or to IgA without passing through IgE first. Note that IgM and IgD are the only two classes that can be concurrently expressed. In addition, since class switching involves deletion of intervening DNA, it cannot be reversed (thus IgG cannot class-switch back to IgM).

    c) Continued binding to antigen is necessary to maintain the survival of plasma cells, and those plasma cells whose mutations confer a higher affinity binding to the stimulating antigen are selected to survive and continue replicating

    d) Clones containing mutations that do not improve the antibody affinity for the antigen are unable to compete for continued antigen binding and die

    e) Affinity maturation occurs concurrently with class switching

    f) **The result is that IgG antibodies are always of significantly higher affinity for the stimulating antigen than were their IgM precursors**

  i. Plasma cells migrate to the bone marrow or mucosa when affinity maturation is complete, and there secrete antibodies into the systemic circulation

j. During generation of plasma cells, memory cells with identical antibody specificities are also formed, which can persist for decades in the host

2. $\alpha\beta$ T Lymphocytes

   a. $\alpha\beta$ refers to the T-cell receptor, which is a dimer of α chains and β chains (see Figure 8.5)

      1) Like antibodies, the variable region of T- cell receptors are generated via recombination of multiple variable DNA segments

      2) Like antibodies, T-cell receptors are regulated by allelic exclusion, so all the T-cell receptors expressed by a given T cell possess identical specificity

      3) **Unlike antibodies, T-cell receptors do not directly bind to stimulating antigen—instead antigen must be "presented" to the T cell in the context of Major Histocompatibility Molecules** (see Figures 8.5 and 8.6)

   b. T cells derive from the bone marrow, but early precursor cells leave the bone marrow and migrate to the thymus for education

      1) In the thymus, autoantigen is presented to maturing T cells in the context of MHC molecules

      2) Those T cells that bind too avidly to the MHC/autoantigen complexes are deemed autoreactive and are induced to undergo apoptosis **(negative selection)**

      3) Those T cells that cannot bind at all to the MHC/autoantigen complexes do not receive a survival signal and undergo apoptosis, while those that bind loosely do receive a survival signal **(positive selection)**

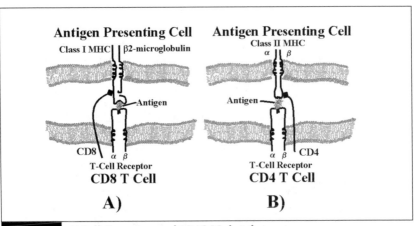

FIGURE 8.5 **T-Cell Receptor and MHC Molecules**

The $\alpha\beta$ T-cell receptor (TCR) is a heterodimer of α and β chains.

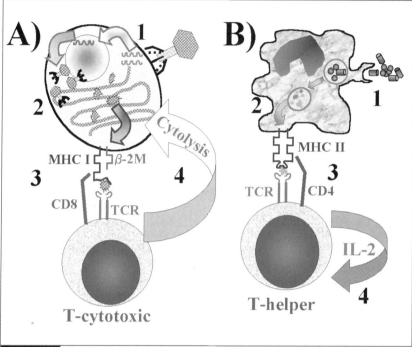

FIGURE 8.6 Antigen Presentation

Antigen presentation to T-cytotoxic (CD8+) and T-helper cells (CD4+). A) 1. A host cell is infected by an intracellular pathogen (virus in this example). 2. As progeny virions are produced, viral antigens are pumped into endoplasmic reticulum where they bind to Class I Major Histocompatibility complex (MHC I) proteins. 3. Covalent interaction with the chaperone protein, β-2 microglobulin, allows surface expression of the MHC I polypeptide, which presents viral antigen bound to a groove at its tip. The CD8 protein on the T-cytotoxic cell binds to the MHC I molecule, stabilizing the interaction between the T-cell receptor (TCR) and the MHC I-antigen complex. 4. The result is activation of the T-cytotoxic cell, which then lyses the host cell to expose the intracellular virus. B) 1. A phagocyte ingests extracellular microbes and degrades them in the phagolysosome. 2. Degraded microbial fragments are loaded onto Class II MHC molecules in the phagolysosome and the MHC II-antigen complexes are transported to the cell surface. 3. CD4 binds to MHC II, stabilizing the interaction between the TCR and the MHC II-antigen complex. 4. The result is activation of the T-helper, which autocrine stimulates its own proliferation by secreting IL-2.

    4) **Result is a T-cell population which has two crucial characteristics**
       a) T cells only respond to antigen presented in the context of MHC molecules (due to positive selection)
       b) T cells do not respond to most self-antigens, even if in the context of MHC molecules (due to negative selection)

c. Also in the thymus, $\alpha\beta$ T cells differentiate to become CD4+ or CD8+
   1) T-cell precursors entering the thymus are double negative (CD4 – CD8–)
   2) Prior to selection, they begin to express both CD8 and CD4, which respectively preferentially bind to Class I and Class II MHC
   3) CD8 ligation of Class I MHC and CD4 ligation of Class II MHC add a certain affinity to the interaction between the T-cell receptor and MHC, which may result in too strong an affinity (negative selection) or just the right affinity (positive selection)
   4) Those T cells positively selected by the combined ligation of the T-cell receptor and CD8 with Class I MHC are induced to shut down expression of CD4, while those positively selected by the T-cell receptor and CD4 binding to Class II MHC are induced to shut down CD8 expression
   5) The result is a population of CD4 – CD8+ T cells restricted to Class I MHC, and CD4+CD8 – T cells restricted to Class II MHC
d. $\alpha\beta$ CD4+ T cells
   1) **These are the classic T-helper cells that regulate immune responses**
   2) After initial activation, they may differentiate into Th1 or Th2 cells (see Figure 8.7)
   3) Th1 cells
      a) Act against small, **phagocytosable, intracellular** pathogens
      b) Characterized by secretion of Interleukin (IL)-2, **Interferon (IFN)**-γ, and Lymphotoxin (LT)-α
      c) Induce potent cell-mediated, inflammatory responses
      d) Antibody stimulation is less marked
      e) Uninhibited Th1 cells are implicated in auto-immunity (e.g., Multiple Sclerosis)
   4) Th2 cells
      a) Act against large, **non-phagocytosable, extracellular** helminths
      b) Characterized by secretion of **IL-4**, IL-5, IL-10, and IL-13
      c) Markedly induce antibody production, also induce class switching to IgE
      d) Act to suppress Th1-mediated inflammatory responses, thereby shifting immune activity from cell-mediated to humoral immunity
      e) Uninhibited Th2 cells implicated in allergic/atopic disorders and asthma
      f) A shift from dominance of Th1 to Th2 cells correlates with progression of AIDS
   5) Th3 cells
      a) Major regulators of mucosal immunity

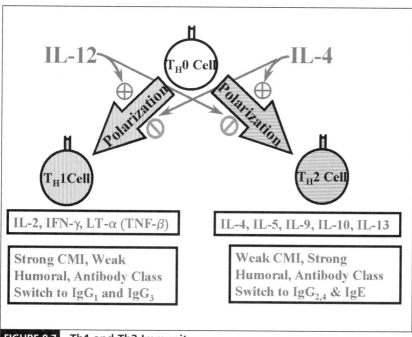

FIGURE 8.7 **Th1 and Th2 Immunity**

Summary of Th1/Th2 induction.

  b) Characterized by high levels of transforming growth factor (TGF)-β production

  c) Induce IgA secretion by B cells

  d) Responsible for Oral Tolerance (see III.B. Tolerance, 5)

 6) CD4+CD25+ T cells

  a) Special T cells that promote tolerance in an antigen specific manner

  b) These cells seem to prevent autoimmunity by contact-induced suppression of other T cells, and by secretion of cytokines such as IL-10 and TGF-β

 e. $\alpha\beta$ CD8+ T cells

  1) **These are cytotoxic T cells (CTLs) that act against viruses and cancers by lysing host cells** (see Figure 8.6)

  2) CTLs expose intracellular pathogens to the immune system by destroying host cells harboring the pathogens

3. $\gamma\delta$ T cells

 a. Express a special T-cell receptor called the $\gamma\delta$ receptor, coded for by entirely separate genes than $\alpha\beta$ receptor

1) $\gamma\delta$ receptor is less polymorphic than $\alpha\beta$ receptor, but is also generated by recombination of variable gene segments
2) Like antibody and unlike the $\alpha\beta$ T-cell receptor, $\gamma\delta$ T-cell receptors can directly bind to certain antigens to become activated

b. Act against evolutionarily conserved antigens in common commensal bacteria and fungi, as well as autoantigens released by necrosed cells (e.g., heat shock proteins)
c. Activated $\gamma\delta$ T cells possess cytotoxic activity akin to CD8 cells, and also secrete a broad range of pro-inflammatory molecules to stimulate the rest of the immune response
d. They are thus presumed to be an evolutionarily primitive (homologues seen in boneless fish) early response element to danger

4. Natural Killer (NK) Lymphocytes
a. Do NOT express T-cell receptor or B-cell receptor
b. **Express inhibitory receptors that bind to Class I MHC molecules, so NK cells are inhibited from killing host cells that express Class I MHC**
c. Certain viruses escape CD8+ T cell-mediated destruction by down-regulating Class I MHC expression by their host cell, but the host cell then becomes susceptible to destruction by NK cells
d. Certain cancers similarly attempt CD8+ T-cell escape and may fall prey to NK cells

IX. MAJOR HISTOCOMPATIBILITY COMPLEX (MHC)

A. General Characteristics

1. **The MHC is responsible for immune recognition of self vs. nonself,** thus organ donation requires matching some or all of the MHC genes from an organ donor with the MHC genes of the recipient—this is the so-called organ "match"

2. MHC genes code for proteins expressed on the surfaces of cells

3. **In humans, MHC proteins are called Human Leukocyte Antigens (HLA)—that is, HLA is synonymous with human MHC**

4. There are six different HLA genes, 3 Class I MHC genes and 3 Class II MHC genes
   a. Human Class I MHC genes are known as HLA-A, HLA-B, and HLA-C
   b. Human Class II MHC genes are known as HLA-DP, HLA-DQ, and HLA-DR

5. **MHC Class I and II are the most polymorphic genes known in humans,** meaning no other genes have been found which have so many different alleles in the population

6. MHC genes are codominant, meaning that each individual expresses one allele of the gene inherited from the mother and one allele of the gene inherited from the father, so each person expresses two alleles of each of the HLA-A, HLA-B, HLA-C, and HLA-DP, HLA-DQ, HLA-DR

7. MHC Class I is expressed by almost every cell in the body, with red blood cells and sperm cells notable exceptions

8. MHC Class II is constitutively expressed only by professional antigen presenting cells
   a. Macrophages, B lymphocytes, and dendritic cells are professional antigen-presenting cells
   b. Endothelial cells can be induced to express Class II MHC by exposure to IFN-γ

9. Certain alleles are linked to disease states
   a. HLA-DR4 (the fourth allele of the Class II MHC gene, HLA-DR) is classically associated with inflammatory arthritic disorders
   b. HLA-B27 (the 27th allele of the Class I gene, HLA-B) is associated with Ankylosing Spondylitis

B. Class I MHC (see Figure 8.6)

1. Utilized to present antigen to CD8+ cytotoxic T cells (CD8 binds to Class I molecule)

2. Transporter of Activating Peptide (TAP) is a pump embedded in the endoplasmic reticulum of all cells, which scavenges the cytoplasm for loose proteins

3. TAP grabs protein fragments generated by the proteasome (a garbage disposal unit which chops up cytoplasmic proteins), and pumps fragments into the endoplasmic reticulum where they bind to Class I MHC molecules

4. Class I MHC molecules loaded with peptides in the endoplasmic reticulum are then transported to the cell surface, where they present the antigen to any T cell passing by

5. **Therefore Class I MHC presents intracellular, cytoplasmic peptides formed from normal cellular metabolism or the metabolism of intracellular pathogens (e.g., viruses, *Chlamydia*, etc.)**

C. Class II MHC (see Figure 8.6)

1. Utilized to present antigen to CD4+ T-helper cells (CD4 binds to Class II molecule)

2. Phagocytic cells degrade ingested particles in the phagolysosome

3. Class II MHC molecules are then transported into the phagolysosome and digested peptides are loaded onto the Class II MHC molecules

4. The peptide-loaded Class II MHC molecules are then transported to the cell surface

5. **Class II MHC presents extracellular antigens, having entered the cell via the phagolysosomal pathway**

D. Transplant Immunology

1. The MHC Match
   a. MHC types of organ donors and organ recipients are checked against one another to find close matches
   b. Each child gets one set of HLA alleles from both parents
   c. HLA genes are co-dominant, so alleles inherited from both parents are expressed in the child
   d. Since both parents also have two sets of alleles (total of four sets between the two parents), and each child gets one set from mom and one set from dad (the child gets two of the four parental

alleles), siblings have a 25% chance of inheriting identical HLA alleles from their parents (1/2 chance of getting same maternal alleles × 1/2 chance of getting same paternal alleles = 1/4 chance of getting same both alleles)

e. On the other hand, since children express both paternal and maternal alleles, they will typically not be matched to either of their parents, unless mom and dad both have identical HLA alleles (a situation only seen with extreme in-breeding)

f. Thus sibling organ donors are the best chance for a perfect HLA match

g. Because of immunosuppressive drugs, perfect matches are not required for successful organ donation, but the more HLA alleles are matched, the better grafts do on average

2. Hyperacute Graft Rejection
   a. Occurs within minutes of transplant
   b. Seen in MHC mismatched recipient who has been previously sensitized to the donor's MHC type (by pregnancy, blood transfusions, prior graft, etc)
   c. Caused by preformed antibodies circulating in recipient's serum
   d. Cannot be reversed, requires removal of graft

3. Acute Graft Rejection
   a. Occurs within weeks of transplant
   b. Seen in MHC mismatched recipient not previously exposed to the donor's MHC type
   c. Caused by CD8+ cytotoxic T cells reacting to foreign MHC molecules
   d. Typically reversible with immunosuppressive agents such as cyclosporin or FK-506, both of which inhibit calcineurin-induced activation of IL-2 secretion from T cells, thereby inhibiting T-cell activation

4. Chronic Graft Rejection
   a. Occurs over months to years after transplant
   b. Caused by antibody damage to vascular system, based upon MHC mismatch
   c. Cannot be reversed with immunosuppressives

X. BASIC CONCEPTS

A. Innate vs. Specific Immunity

1. Innate Immunity
   a. Skin
      1) Serves as a structural barrier against microbial entry into the host
      2) Also colonized by commensal organisms which compete for nutrients thereby inhibiting growth of pathogens
   b. Mucous membranes
      1) **Bathed in fluids containing lysozyme,** an enzyme which lyses bacterial cell walls
      2) **Mucosal fluids also contain high concentration of secretory IgA,** which blocks microbial adhesion to mucosal epithelium
      3) Covered with cilia that sweep away particulates and microbes
   c. Chemical barriers
      1) The body uses toxic pH levels in the stomach to protect the GI tract, and pH levels in the dermis and vagina inhibit overgrowth of bacteria
      2) **Chelation of iron during inflammation is a very potent inhibitor of microbial growth,** explaining why iron-binding proteins such as transferrin and ferritin go up during inflammation (so-called acute phase reactants)
   d. Phagocytes (from the Greek "phago" = eat, "cyte" = cell, "phagocyte" = eater cell)
      1) Neutrophils, monocyte/macrophages, eosinophils, and dendritic cells are professional phagocytes
      2) Phagocytes migrate through the peripheral vasculature and are recruited into tissue at the start of an inflammatory response
         a) **Recruitment begins with local elicitation of chemotactic cytokines, called chemokines, secreted by injured cells** or by stressed cells neighboring the injured cells
         b) Chemokines diffuse into the bloodstream, setting up a concentration gradient allowing phagocytes to home-in on the source
         c) Chemokines, as well as bacterial antigens such as endotoxin, also activate the phagocytes, causing them to express adhesion molecules on their surface
      3) When phagocytes reach the source of the chemokine gradient, they undergo a **three-step process known as extravasation,** allowing them to leave the vasculature and enter peripheral tissue (see Figure 10.1)

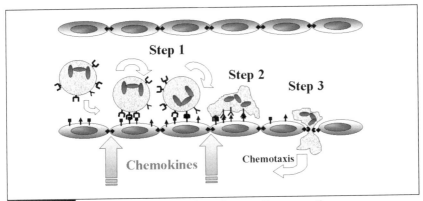

FIGURE 10.1   Three-Step Model of Leukocyte Extravasation

Leukocyte extravasation from the intravascular compartment into parenchyma is a three-step process. Step 1) Inflammatory cytokines released at the site of infection induce endothelial cells to express selectin molecules on their cell surface (⊤). Chemokines diffuse from the site of infection into the blood stream, creating a concentration gradient to attract leukocytes from the intravascular compartment. Such chemokines also induce leukocytes to express selectin-ligands on their cell surface (Ψ). Leukocytes following the chemokine gradient migrate toward the endothelium neighboring the site of infection and the low affinity interaction between selectins and selectin-ligands results in rolling of the leukocyte along the endothelium. Step 2) Binding of selectins to selectin-ligands induces higher affinity adhesions, such as ICAM (v) on endothelial cells and LFA (+) on leukocytes, to be expressed. These higher affinity interactions cause the leukocytes to cease rolling and firmly adhere to the endothelium. Step 3) Freed from the shear forces of blood flow, the leukocytes crawl across the endothelium and diapedese between the endothelial cells, disrupting the binding of PECAM-PECAM homodimers which hold neighboring endothelial cells together (••). The leukocytes unzip the PECAM homodimers and use the PECAM molecules on either side as traction to propel the leukocytes out of the blood vessel and into tissue. Subsequently the leukocytes crawl through the tissue along the chemokine concentration gradient, leading back to the site of infection.

a) **Step 1**: binding to selectin molecules on the endothelial cells causes the phagocyte to roll along the inner wall of the blood vessel
b) **Step 2**: binding to **ICAM** causes the phagocyte to stop rolling and firmly **adhere** to the endothelium
c) **Step 3**: the phagocyte undergoes **diapedesis**, squeezing in between the endothelial cells and binding to PECAM at the endothelial cell junction, allowing it to crawl out of the blood vessel toward the source of the chemokines

4) Phagocytosis is triggered by binding of one of several receptors on the phagocyte to its target ligand
   a) **The phagocyte Fcγ receptor binds to the constant regions (Fc) of IgG antibodies (γ = IgG, thus Fcγ = receptor for the Fc of IgG)** allowing ingestion of any particle attached to the antibody variable region
   b) The phagocyte Complement Receptor 3 (CR3) binds to complement fragments deposited on microbes
   c) **Phagocyte Toll-family receptors bind directly to conserved elements in microbial cell walls,** such as gram negative lipopolysaccharide (endotoxin)
5) Following phagocytosis, the phagosome fuses with lysosomes and neutrophil or eosinophil granules, the contents of which mediate killing of any microbes in the phagolysosome
6) Phagocytosis also stimulates the leukocyte to undergo the respiratory or oxidative burst
   a) NADPH oxidase assembles on the phagosome membrane, generating superoxide anion (O_2^-) from oxygen
   b) Superoxide is converted to one of a variety of toxic metabolites
      i) Superoxide dismutase converts the superoxide to hydrogen peroxide (H_2O_2), which has intrinsic antimicrobial properties
      ii) **In neutrophils, myeloperoxidase combines peroxide with chloride anions to generate hypochlorite** (HClO– common house bleach) which is highly toxic to microbes in the phagosome
7) **Importance of phagocytes demonstrated by the markedly elevated risk of death from infection in neutropenic patients**

e. Fever
   1) **Fever is a host response to infection**
   2) **Systemic IL-1, IL-6, or TNF, generated in response to bacterial pyrogens such as lipopolysaccharide, cause the hypothalamic thermostat to reset higher**
   3) Growth of some microbes is optimized to normal body temperature, and fever results in a partial inhibition of their growth
   4) Phagocytosis and the respiratory burst are more efficient at higher temperatures

f. Complement (see Figure 10.2)
   1) A reactive cascade of serum proteins resulting in three beneficial effects
      a) The generation of protein fragments chemotactic for leukocytes (e.g., C3a and C5a)

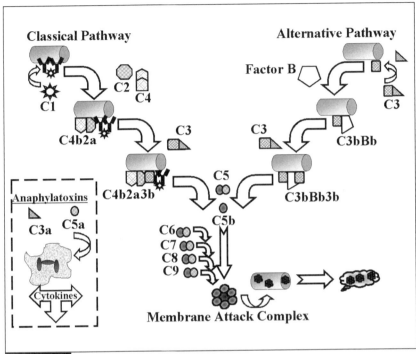

FIGURE 10.2 The Complement Cascade

The complement cascade can be initiated by binding of C1 to the Fc domains of antibody (the Classical Pathway), or by direct binding of C3 to microbial glycolipids (the Alternative Pathway). See text for a description of each component in the cascade.

b) **Opsonization** (from the Greek for "to make palatable"), or the coating of microbes with host protein fragments (e.g., C3b) that enable phagocytosis

c) Generation of the **membrane attack complex** (MAC, comprised of C5 to C8), which punches holes in microbial cell membranes

2) The complement components C1 to C4 have **serine protease activity**, activating the next component in the cascade by cleaving the next component in two, thereby exposing the active enzyme site of that next component

3) At each step along the cascade, enzymatic serine protease activity results in significant amplification of the response, meaning that activation of one molecule of a complement component leads to activation of hundreds or thousands of the next molecule in the cascade

    4) There are two pathways to activate the complement cascade
      a) The Classical Pathway
          i)   **The constant region of antibodies,** or acute phase reactants such as C-reactive protein, bind to C1, bringing it in close proximity to a microbe
          ii) C1 acts as a serine protease to cleave C2 and C4, forming C4b2a
          iii) C4b2a is known as C3 convertase, because it cleaves thousands of copies of C3 into C3a and C3b
          iv) C3a is known as an anaphylatoxin because it binds to mast cells and basophils and stimulates massive release of histamine, generating local inflammation
          v)   C3b deposited onto microbes opsonizes them, allowing binding of phagocytes via the CR3 receptor
          vi) C3b also joins C4b2a to form C4b2a3b, which converts C5 to C5a and C5b
          vii) Like C3a, C5a is also an anaphylatoxin, while C5b initiates the membrane attack complex formation by successive binding of C6, C7, C8, and C9
          viii) The membrane attack complex punches a donut-shaped hole in the microbial cell membrane, resulting in osmotic lysis
      b) The Alternative Pathway
          i)   **C3 can directly bind to evolutionarily conserved microbial surface antigens**
          ii) This results in spontaneous degradation of C3 to C3a and C3b
          iii) Factor B binds to C3b and is then cleaved by Factor D, forming C3bBb
          iv) C3bBb is analogous to C4b2a3b of the Classical Pathway, acting as a C5 convertase
          v)   **Thus, the Alternative and Classical Pathways are initiated by different mechanisms, but have in common every step from C5 convertase forward**
  g. Cytokines also have innate immune functions, particularly IL-1 and interferons (see cytokines section)

2. Specific Immunity
  a. **Specificity is provided to immune responses ONLY via B and T lymphocytes**
  b. Specificity of lymphocytes is dependent upon their antigen receptors, which are created during cellular ontogeny by gene recombination events
  c. Unlike innate immunity, specific immunity has memory: the specific immune system responds differently the second time it sees the same antigen/microbe

d. **Memory**
   1) Memory lymphocytes differentiate following the initial, primary immune response mediated by a particular lymphocyte
   2) Memory cells are long-lived, and continue to re-circulate throughout the body until they again encounter the same antigen that initiated the primary response
   3) **Memory cells are responsible for two important clinical effects**
      a) Vaccination is possible by stimulation of high levels of memory cells
      b) Infections like chicken pox rarely occur twice in the same person due to memory cells induced following the first infection
e. Primary versus Secondary Immunity
   1) A primary immune response results the first time lymphocytes are activated against a given antigen
   2) Secondary immune responses occur following reactivation of memory cells generated during the primary response
   3) Secondary immunity is faster, more powerful and more specific

B. Tolerance

1. **Tolerance is the lack of immune responses against self-tissues (lack of autoimmunity)**
2. **Since only lymphocytes are specific effectors, tolerance is dependent upon lymphocytic functions**
3. Two general mechanisms of tolerance are Central and Peripheral
   a. Central Tolerance
      1) **Provided by T-cell education during development in the thymus**
      2) As described above, immature T-cells which are strongly reactive to self-tissues, undergo negative selection and are induced to apoptose in the thymus
      3) **Central tolerance is imperfect because it is impossible to expose the lymphocytes in the thymus to every possible antigen contained within the human body**
   b. Peripheral Tolerance
      1) **Acts as a crucial backup to central tolerance**
      2) Four major mechanisms of peripheral tolerance
         a) Previously mentioned CD4+CD25+ T cells suppress other T-cell activities
         b) **Antigenic ignorance**
            i) If T cells never see certain self-antigens (called cryptic antigens), they can never respond to them even if they are capable of doing so

      ii)   Significant portions of parenchymal organs are never exposed to the immune system unless they are damaged by trauma or inflammation

      iii) Arthritis and diabetes may be examples of diseases where trauma or infection damages tissue, exposing T cells to cryptic antigens against which they have not been centrally tolerized, initiating autoimmunity

  c) **Co-stimulation** (Two-Signal Lymphocyte Activation)

      i)   **Like B cells, all $\alpha\beta$ T cells (CD4+ and CD8+) require two signals for activation**

      ii)   Professional phagocytes act as antigen presenting cells, complexing ingested antigen with MHC molecules to present to T cells (Signal 1)

      iii) However, professional phagocytes also must provide a second signal to enable T-cell activation

      iv) The second signal can be provided by co-stimulatory ligand binding, the most famous of which is B7 on the antigen-presenting cell binding to CD28 on the T cell

      v)   **In general, phagocytes only provide the second signal for stimulation when the phagocyte recognizes danger in the environment**

          a)) Danger is recognized by phagocytes when they are exposed to evolutionarily conserved microbial fragments, such as gram negative lipopolysaccharide, gram positive cell wall lipotechoic acid, or prokaryotic DNA, each of which can bind to specific receptors on the phagocyte

          b)) Danger is also recognized by phagocytes when they are exposed to inflammatory cytokines provided by early response elements of the innate immune system (e.g., neutrophils or damaged parenchymal cells leaking IL-1)

      vi) Phagocytes recognizing danger signals undergo activation, and are thus primed to provide a second signal to activate T-cells, but phagocytes that have not recognized a danger signal are presumed to be presenting antigens from non-threatening particulates which might in fact be host proteins

      vii) Thus the second signal requirement is a fail-safe to prevent activation of potentially auto-reactive T cells

      viii) **T cells receiving Signal 1 (MHC/antigen binding to T-cell receptor) without Signal 2 become either anergic (tolerized to the antigen for which they are specific) or they apoptose**

  d) Oral Tolerance

      i)   Induced by Th3 cells due to ↑ TGF-β production

ii) Can induce tolerance to otherwise immunogenic proteins by feeding them to people
iii) TGF-β anergizes otherwise reactive T-cells in the gut mucosa
iv) Failure of Oral Tolerance leads to Inflammatory Bowel Disease

C. Autoimmunity

1. Due to aberrant lymphocyte (mostly T cell) responses caused by breakage of tolerance
2. Several mechanisms of autoimmunity are known
   a. Reversal of antigenic ignorance
      1) Occurs when inflammation develops in parenchymal tissues
      2) Tissue destruction exposes T cells to autoantigens that had previously been sequestered (so called "cryptic antigens")
      3) T cells potentially reactive to cryptic antigens are not deleted because such antigens are not expressed in the thymus
      4) Since inflammation is ongoing, phagocytes will be exposed to danger signals in the form of inflammatory cytokines, and can present autoantigens to T cells along with a second signal, causing T-cell activation
   b. **Molecular Mimicry**
      1) T cells are activated against microbes which have antigens structurally similar to self-antigens
      2) As the immune system revs up, it becomes confused and attacks both the microbe and the self-tissue
      3) Example: rheumatic fever involves immune response to heart valve proteins similar to antigens found in *Streptococcus*
   c. Aberrant cytokine regulation
      1) Out-of-control Th1 or Th2 responses lead to self-destruction
      2) Causes of the loss of control are unclear in most instances
      3) Examples
         a) Th1: tuberculosis and hepatitis kill people due to inflammatory response, not due to direct effects of the microbe/virus
         b) Th2: allergy, asthma, anaphylaxis

XI. CYTOKINES—A BRIEF GUIDE*

*Cytokines in **boldface** are most likely to appear on board exams.

TABLE 11.1	Cytokines	
CYTOKINE	**CHARACTERISTICS**	**FUNCTIONS**
IL-1 α/β	**Immediate danger signals,** released when cells are damaged—also induces fever	• Initiate inflammation • Endogenous pyrogen
IL-2	**Required for T-cell proliferation**	• T-cell proliferation
IL-3	Stem cell growth factor	• Stem cell growth factor
IL-4	Stimulates antibody production, linked to atopy and asthma, made by Th2 cells	• Stimulates antibody secretion • Stimulates IgE class switch
IL-5	Eosinophil growth and activation factor, also implicared in asthma/atopy	• Important in IgE response • Anti-parasite host defense
IL-6	Systemic marker of inflammation, stimulates acute phase reactants	• Endogenous pyrogen • Acute phase reactant
IL-7	Growth/survival factor for lymphocytes	• Lymphocyte growth factor
IL-8	Chemotactic for neutrophils	• Neutrophil chemoattractant
IL-9	Growth and survival factor for mast cells	• Mast cell growth factor
IL-10	Inhibits expression of almost all cytokines, suppresses inflammation	• General immunosuppressive
IL-11	Stimulates platelet formation, is also anti-inflammatory and ↑ iron absorption in the gut may explain why platelets ↑ in chronic inflammation and iron deficiency	• Stimulates platelet production • Suppresses inflammation • ↑ iron absorption in the gut
IL-12	Produced by antigen presenting cells, induces Th1 differentiation	• Induces Th1 differentiation

TABLE 11.1	*Continued*	
CYTOKINE	**CHARACTERISTICS**	**FUNCTIONS**
IL-13	Mimics IL-4 functions	• Stimulates antibody secretion • Stimulates IgE class switch
IL-14	May be a B-cell growth factor	• ? B-cell growth factor
IL-15	Mimics IL-2 functions	• T-cell growth factor
IL-16	Chemotactic for CD4 T cells	• Chemotactic for CD4 T cells
IL-17	Non-specific inflammatory stimulator	• Stimulates inflammation
IL-18	Induces production of IFN-γ	• Induces IFN-γ production
IFN-α	Induces anti-viral state in parenchymal cells by altering surface receptors and turning on cellular RNAses and DNAses to chop up invading RNA and DNA	• Induces antiviral state • Activates phagocytes
IFN-β	Secreted by fibroblasts, role unclear in vivo, ? feedback suppression	• ? feedback suppression from inflammation
IFN-γ	Induces antiviral state, markedly stimulates phagocytic activity and Th1 induction	• Induces antiviral state • Stimulates inflammation
TNF	Non-specific inflammatory mediator, endogenous pyrogen, causes cachexia	• Stimulates inflammation • Causes cachexia (formerly called cachectin)
Lympho-toxin-α	Secreted only by Th1 cells, induces apoptosis in target cells, stimulates inflammation	• Induces apoptosis • Stimulates inflammation
TGF-β	Terminates immune responses, induces antigen-specific anergy in T cells, stimulates IgA secretion, causes fibrosis, responsible for oral tolerance	• Causes class switching to IgA • Regulates mucosal immunity • Causes oral tolerance • Causes fibrosis
G-CSF	Stimulates granulocyte production, utilized clinically for neutropenia (Neupogen)	• Stimulates granulocyte production
GM-CSF	Stimulates granulocyte and monocyte production	• Stimulates granulocyte and monocyte production

XII. IMMUNE ORGAN SYSTEMS

A. Primary Immune Organs (sites of immune cell progenitors)

1. Bone Marrow
   a. The primary hematopoietic organ in the adult human
   b. Possess stem cells which respond to growth factor signals by differentiating into all of the different types of blood
   c. **Also harbors active antibody-producing B cells (plasma cells)**

2. Thymus
   a. Secretes cytokines chemotactic for T lymphocyte precursor cells, which leave the bone marrow and migrate to the thymus
   b. Structurally composed of an outer cortex and inner medulla
   c. Cortex
      1) Newly arrived T cells disembark in the subcapsular zone above the cortex, and then migrate down into the cortex
      2) During their migration through the cortex, immature T cells interact with thymic epithelial cells expressing Class I and Class II MHC molecules
      3) **Positive selection occurs here**—that is, only those immature T cells whose receptors are capable of binding to MHC molecules expressed on the thymic cortical epithelium are given survival signals, while T cells with receptors incapable of binding to MHC molecules undergo apoptosis
      4) The positively selected T cells then migrate deeper into the cortex toward the medulla
   d. Medulla
      1) The medulla is populated by bone-marrow derived macrophages and dendritic cells
      2) As the maturing, positively selected T cells migrate to the medulla, they interact with these macrophages and dendritic cells, which also express Class I and Class II MHC molecules
      3) Those positively selected T cells that interact too strongly with the MHC molecules on the macrophages and dendritic cells are given a death signal, forcing them to undergo apoptosis
      4) **Thus, negative selection occurs in the thymic medulla**, eliminating potentially autoreactive T cells that survived positive selection in the cortex
      5) **99% of T cells entering the thymus undergo apoptosis**, while 1% migrate out of the medulla to enter systemic circulation

B. Secondary Immune Organs (sites of initiation of immune responses)

1. Lymph Nodes (see Figure 12.1)
   a. Aggregations of immune cells placed along lymph channels

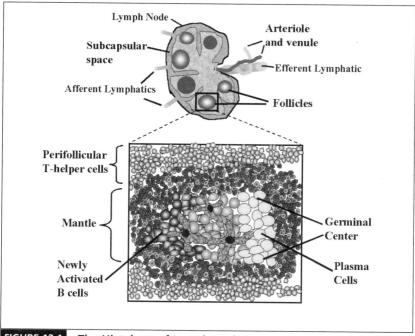

FIGURE 12.1 The Histology of Lymph Nodes

A lymph node is shown in cross-section, with a magnified image of a secondary follicle. Primary follicles have no germinal center (no central clearing). Secondary follicles have a germinal center, in which large, proliferating B cells are exposed to antigen presented by dendritic cells. Affinity maturation and class switching occur in the germinal centers. In the figure, newly activated B lymphocytes occupy the left-most portion of the germinal center. These cells migrate to the right as they divide, brushing against the follicular dendritic cells, which expose the B cells to antigen in order to further drive affinity to maturation and class switching. At the right side of the germinal center are mature effector B cells, called plasma cells, which secrete high-affinity IgG antibodies. From the germinal centers these activated, antibody-secreting cells will migrate into the efferent lymph channel, and from there to bone marrow, submucosa, or spleen to secrete their antibodies into the circulation. A rim of darkly staining B lymphocytes, known as the follicular mantle, surrounds the germinal center. Outside the mantle are CD4+ T-helper cells, occupying the perifollicular areas.

    b. Lymph channels drain interstitial fluid from epithelial and parenchymal tissues, routing such fluid back into the vascular compartment via the thoracic duct

    c. In addition, lymph carries antigenic materials floating about in the interstitial fluid to the lymph nodes for sampling by immune cells

    d. **Thus, lymph nodes are designed like filters, allowing the detritus of host and foreign tissues to be accumulated and sifted through by host defense cells**

    e. Like the thymus, lymph nodes can be separated into cortex and medulla

    f. Cortex

       1) The cortex contains multiple follicles, which are masses of B lymphocytes and dendritic cells jammed together

       2) **Follicles without germinal centers are known as primary follicles, while those containing germinal centers are known as secondary follicles**

       3) **Germinal centers are the result of massive B-lymphocyte proliferation following activation, and are the locations where class switching and affinity maturation occurs during B-cell activation**

       4) T cells occupy the parafollicular areas, which separate the follicles

    g. Medulla

       1) Sparsely populated by migrating lymphocytes and macrophages

       2) This is where the vasculature penetrates the node

       3) Specialized endothelial cells, called High Endothelial Venules, express adhesion molecules allowing lymphocytes to extravasate across the venules in order to migrate into the lymph node

2. Spleen

    a. Analogous to the lymph nodes filtering lymph of antigen, **the spleen is a giant filter trap for particulate antigens in the vascular compartment**

    b. Red pulp

       1) Comprises areas dominated by red blood cells and macrophages

       2) Arterioles course off the splenic artery, ending in open sinuses surrounded by macrophages

       3) Macrophages ingest particulate matter in the blood, and also destroy senescent red cells

    c. White pulp

       1) Comprised of areas dominated by lymphocytes

2) Arterioles are surrounded by cuffs of lymphocytes (the periar-teriolar lymphoid sheaths, or PALS), which form follicles akin to lymph node follicles

3. Mucosal Associated Lymphoid Tissues (MALT)
   a. Organized lymphoid tissues found interspersed along the gas-trointestinal and respiratory tracts
   b. Follicles form in the submucosa, akin to lymph node follicles
   c. Th3 cells predominate in MALT, causing B cell class-switching to IgA
   d. In the gastrointestinal tract, specialized epithelial cells known as M cells sample the intestinal lumen by endocytosing particulate matter, process the matter and present it as antigen to underly-ing lymphocytes

XIII. HYPERSENSITIVITY REACTIONS

A. Allergic Hypersensitivity (Type 1)

1. IgE-mediated, due to release of vasoactive mediators from mast cells and basophils
   a. Following initial exposure to allergen, anti-allergen B cells are induced to class switch to IgE in the presence of IL-4
   b. Secreted IgE circulates in the vasculature and binds to receptors on mast cells and basophils which are specific for the constant region of the IgE (Fcε receptors)
   c. Upon re-exposure of the allergen, the IgE antibodies sitting on the mast cell and basophil surfaces are cross-linked, causing the cells
   to degranulate, spilling histamine and leukotrienes into the vasculature

2. Examples = allergies, anaphylaxis, atopic diseases

B. Cytotoxic Hypersensitivity (Type 2)

1. Antibody-mediated, typically IgG binds to antigen on target cell surface, inducing complement lysis, ADCC, or phagocytosis

2. Examples = autoimmune hemolytic anemia, Erythroblastosis Fetalis, pemphigus, Goodpasture's Disease, penicillin-induced anemia, hyperacute transplant rejection

C. Immune Complex Hypersensitivity (Type 3, Arthus Reaction)

1. In the presence of high titer, high affinity IgG antibody, antigens in the serum are bound into large complexes cross-linked by multiple antibodies

2. These large antigen-antibody complexes circulate through the vasculature, and although some are cleared by macrophages in the spleen, some of the complexes deposit in epithelial crevices throughout the body

3. Deposited antigen-antibody complexes bind complement, which attracts neutrophils and induces lytic enzyme release, causing tissue damage

4. Examples = serum sickness, SLE systemic findings, post-infectious glomerulonephritis

D. Delayed Type Hypersensitivity (DTH, Type 4)

1. Induction of Th1 responses causes the local accumulation of phagocytes

2. This response is dependent upon IFN-γ secreted by Th1 cells

3. The result is organized cell-mediated immunity, typified by granulomatous reaction in the subcutaneous or intra-dermal tissues

4. Examples = contact dermatitis, acute/chronic transplant rejection, TB, and poison ivy

XIV. IMMUNODEFICIENCIES

A. Primary Immunodeficiencies

TABLE 14.1	B-Lymphocyte Deficiencies	
• Recurrent encapsulated bacterial infections in infants >6 months old		
• Diagnosis often made by Quantitative Immunoglobulin Analysis (QUIG), revealing abnormal levels of serum immunoglobulin (Ig) subtypes		
DISEASE	**PATHOPHYSIOLOGY**	**PRESENTATION**
Bruton's Agamma-globulinemia	• X-linked defect of tyrosine kinase causes defective B cell development	• Always male patients (X-linked) • **No B cells in blood** (normal # of precursors in marrow) • Pts are treated with IVIG
Hyper-IgM Syndrome	• CD40 defect prevents IgG class switching	• QUIG → normal levels of IgM but no IgG • Pts are treated with IVIG
Selective Ig Deficiency	• IgA deficiency most common primary immunodeficiency affects 1/600 Caucasians (can also have IgG deficiency) • Caused by defects in isotype class switching	• Affected people have **recurrent sinus and respiratory infections, chronic diarrhea, and asthma**, although may be asymptomatic • IgG deficiency causes bronchiectasis • IgA deficient pts (who do have IgG) have anaphylactoid reactions to IgA contained in blood products, **so do not Tx with IVIG** • QUIG → ↓ IgA (or IgG) but normal numbers of peripheral B cells
Common Variable Hypogamma-globulinemia	• An **acquired** defect • Causes ↓ IgG production due to defect in plasma cell differentiation	• Recurrent encapsulated bacterial infections **in patients aged 15–35, with splenomegaly and lymphadenopathy** • QUIG → ↓ antibody levels in the face of normal B cell counts • Treat with monthly IVIG

TABLE 14.2	**T-Lymphocyte Deficiencies**	
• Recurrent severe viral, fungal, or protozoal infections from infancy		
• QUIG → normal IgM levels but ↓ IgG and IgA due to defective class switching		
DISEASE	**PATHOPHYSIOLOGY**	**PRESENTATION**
DiGeorge's Syndrome	• Embryological defect in pharyngeal pouch 3 and 4 → thymic aplasia which cases T-cell deficiency, and parathyroid aplasia	• **Presents with tetany due to hypocalcemia 2° to hypoparathyroidism** • **Syndromic facies (micrognathia, short philtrum), and congenital cardiac defects** • ↓ CD4 and CD8 T cells
Ataxia-Telangiectasia	• Autosomal recessive defect in DNA repair • Causes thymic dysfunction • B cells develop normally	• **Truncal ataxia in infancy, telangiectasias, recurrent repiratory infxns → bronchiectasis** • Pts should avoid radiation due to very high risk of lymphoma and carcinoma • ↓ CD4 and CD8 T cells
Bare Lymphocyte Syndrome	• Lack of Class II MHC prevents positive selection of CD4 T cells in the thymus	• Labs → ↓ CD4 T cells in blood, but normal number of CD8 cells

B. Acquired

1. Acquired Immunodeficiency Syndrome (AIDS)—see Microbiology Section V.B.2.a.3)a)
2. Drug Induced
   a. Corticosteroids
      1) The most immunosuppressive drugs available
      2) Simultaneously suppress T-cell, B-cell, and phagocyte functions
      3) Multiple mechanisms of action, including suppression of pro-inflammatory cytokines, suppression of T-cell activation, suppression of phagocytosis, suppression of oxidative burst and intracellular killing, and possibly direct induction of lymphocyte death
      4) Make patient susceptible to all types of infections, including typical pyogenic bacteria, opportunistic bacteria (i.e., *Listeria*,

TABLE 14.3	Combined B- and T-Lymphocyte Deficiencies	
DISEASE	**PATHOPHYSIOLOGY**	**PRESENTATION**
Severe Combined Immuno-Deficiency (SCID)	• Due to variety of metabolic or cytokine receptor defects, these are the classic "bubble boy" patients • Can be autosomal recessive, X-linked, or sporadic	• **Viral, bacterial, fungal, and protozoal infections, children get sick within weeks of birth** • Bone marrow transplantation has met with moderate success • Blood transfusions can cause Graft Versus Host Disease (GVHD)
Wiskott-Aldrich Syndrome	• X-linked recessive defect in IgM production to capsular polysaccharides • Also poorly characterized T-cell defects	QUIG → ↓ IgM, Nml IgG, ↑ **IgA and IgE**, B cell # normal, T cells anergic • **Classic Triad: eczema, pyogenic bacterial infections, and thrombocytopenia, always in males** • Leukemia and lymphoma is common in children who survive to 10 years old • First line Tx is BMT, second line is IVIG

atypical *Mycobacteria, Nocardia,* etc.), opportunistic fungi (i.e., *Pneumocystis, Aspergillus*), parasites (i.e., *Strongyloides*), and even viruses (i.e., CMV)

  b. Cyclosporine and FK506

    1) Chief mechanism of action is inhibition of calcineurin, a key signal transducer active following ligation of the T-cell receptor

    2) Hence, these drugs chiefly suppress T-cell function, leaving all other arms of the immune system relatively intact

    3) Very potent at preventing graft rejection, but much less prone to make patients susceptible to infection, although risk for opportunistic organisms like *Pneumocystis* are still increased

TABLE 14.4	**Phagocyte Deficiencies**	

• Recurrent bacterial infections, usually catalase ⊕ (e.g., *Staph*), also *Aspergillus*

DISEASE	PATHOPHYSIOLOGY	PRESENTATION
Chronic Granulomatous Disease	• Phagocytes lack respiratory burst, can engulf microbes but are unable to kill them	• Lab → defective O_2^-/H_2O_2 production by phagocytes • Infections often caused by *S. aureus* or *Aspergillus* • Tx = Recombinant IFN-γ
Leukocyte Adhesion Deficiency Syndromes	• Type I due to lack of β_2-integrins (LFA-1) • Type II due to lack of selectin receptors	• **Gingivitis, poor wound healing, and delayed umbilical cord separation** caused because neutrophils can't extravasate into tissues
Chédiak-Higashi Syndrome	• Autosomal recessive defect of microtubule function of neutrophils → inability to fuse lysosomes and phagosome	• Present with recurrent infections with *Staph* and *Strep*, **albinism**, peripheral and cranial neuropathies • Lab: giant granules seen in PMN on blood smear
Job's Syndrome (Hyper-IgE)	• High IgE levels and inhibition of neutrophil chemotaxis	• **"Cold"** *Staph* abscesses and respiratory infections, **double rows of teeth** in jaw, brittle bones, **classic "gargoyle facies"** • Lab: IgE > 2000 mg/dL (Nml < 500)

TABLE 14.5	Complement Deficiencies	
DISEASE	**PATHOPHYSIOLOGY**	**PRESENTATION**
Hereditary Angioedema	• Deficiency of C1 esterase inhibitor, so C1 continues to generate vasoactive C3a and C5a, causing ↑ capillary permeability and edema	• Brawny edema of face and mouth, and **if edema of supraglottis occurs this can cause fatal airway obstruction** • Tx = ↑ C1 inhibitor concentration with Danazol, or ↓ C1 activation with ε-amino-caproic acid (inhibits plasminogen) • Airway observation
C1, C2, or C4 Deficiency	• Defect in clearance of antigen/antibody complexes	• Present with lupus-like autoimmune disorder, also pyogenic infxn in some
C3 or C5 Deficiency	• Blocks both alternative and classical complement pathways	• Recurrent pyogenic bacterial infections, typically *Staphylococcus*
C6, C7, C8, or C9 Deficiency	• Blocks development of Membrane Attack Complex	• **Classic presentation is recurrent *Neisseria* infections** • Recrudescent *N. meningitidis* meningitis is highly suggestive

XV. TESTABLE LABORATORY IMMUNOLOGY

A. Mitogens

1. Mitogens are inducers of mitosis (mitosis + genic = mitogen)

2. Exposure of immune cells to mitogens induces their activation in a polyclonal fashion—that is, all B cells exposed to a B-cell mitogen are activated irrespective of their particular antigen specificity

B. Enzyme-Linked Immunosorbent Assay (ELISA)

1. Used to measure the amount of antigen or antibody in solution

2. ELISAs use antibody chemically linked to a color-generating enzyme to measure the quantity of antigen or antibody in solution

3. Direct ELISA detects the concentration of antigen in solution

   a. An antibody directed against the antigen of interest is adsorbed onto a plastic plate

   b. A solution containing the antigen of interest is poured onto the plate and incubated, allowing binding of the antigen to the antibody

   c. A second antibody directed against a different epitope on the antigen is linked to a color-generating enzyme, and then added to the plate

   d. After adding the enzymes substrate, the optical density of color generated in the plate can be used to measure the concentration of enzyme present, and thus the concentration of antigen present

TABLE 15.1 Mitogens	
MITOGEN	**AFFECTED CELL**
Lipopolysaccharide	B cell only
Concanavalin A (con A)	T cell only
Phytohemagglutinin (PHA)	T cell only
Pokeweed Mitogen (PWM)	B and T cells
Superantigens*	T cell only

*Superantigens are toxins that bind non-specifically to T-cell receptors outside the normal antigen-binding cleft, allowing activation of up to 1/5 of all the T cells in the body at any one time.

4. The indirect ELISA is used to measure the concentration of antibody in serum (this is, for example, the type of ELISA which detects anti-HIV antibodies in human serum)

   a. Antigen to which the antibody of interest binds is adsorbed onto a plastic plate (e.g., to assay for anti-HIV antibodies, HIV proteins are adsorbed onto a plate)

   b. Serum is poured onto the plate and incubated, allowing binding of the antibody of interest to the adsorbed antigen

   c. An enzyme-linked anti-antibody antibody, which binds to the constant region of all IgG molecules, is added to the plate

   d. After adding the enzyme substrate, the concentration of antibody present on the plate can be estimated by measuring the color density generated by the enzyme

C. Western Blot

1. A group of proteins (or serum) is electrophoretically run out on a polyacrylamide gel (PAGE)

2. An antibody that recognizes the protein of interest is tagged with an enzyme that generates a visible color, or with a radiation label, and is added to the gel

3. The presence of the protein of interest is inferred from the generation of a colored line or a radioactive signal on the gel at the right molecular weight for the protein of interest

4. The Western Blot is technically more demanding than the ELISA, but in certain circumstances is more accurate

5. For this reason, in AIDS testing all positive ELISAs are confirmed by Western Blotting

D. Monoclonal Antibodies

1. Repeated immunizations in mice cause the generation of memory B lymphocytes, which generate antibody against the antigen used

2. The spleen of the immunized mouse is removed and B cells are isolated

3. The B cells are mixed with immortal myeloma cells that do not secrete antibody, and the two cell types are induced to fuse together by addition of a special chemical—this generates a hybridoma, a cell containing the chromosomes of both the B lymphocyte and the myeloma cell

4. The hybridomas are grown in a special medium that poisons unfused cells so they cannot grow

5. The hybridomas are thus selected to grow out, and after separating into individual wells, their supernatants can be assayed for the presence of a desired antibody

6. In this way, an immortal hybridoma is generated that produces an antibody of a single specificity, and can be used to generate an unlimited amount of that antibody

IMMUNOLOGY REVIEW

QUESTIONS

1. Which of the following is the fundamental function of antibody-dependent cell-mediated cytotoxicity (ADCC)?
   a) Antibody directly kills foreign microbes
   b) Antibody attaches to the B-cell surface, causing the B cell to undergo apoptosis
   c) The Fc portion of antibody attaches to the T-cell surface, and the variable portion provides specificity to T-cell–mediated killing
   d) The Fc portion of antibody attaches to the phagocytic cell surface, and the variable portion provides specificity to phagocyte-mediated killing
   e) Antibody directly kills host lymphocytes

2. Which of the following is not considered part of the differential diagnosis of eosinophilia?
   a) Infection caused by *Coccidioides immitis*
   b) Infection caused by *Candida albicans*
   c) Infection caused by *Trichinella*
   d) Non-Hodgkin's lymphoma
   e) Systemic lupus erythematosus

3. Which of the following cell types do not express Class II MHC molecules?
   a) Macrophages
   b) B lymphocytes
   c) Dendritic cells
   d) T lymphocytes
   e) Endothelial cells

4. An antibody is composed of . . .
   a) 2 heavy chains and 2 light chains.
   b) 2 heavy chains and 1 light chain.
   c) 4 heavy chains and 1 light chain.
   d) 4 heavy chains and 2 light chains.
   e) 4 heavy chains and 4 light chains.

5. Match the following classes of antibody with their functions:
   1) IgM
   2) IgD
   3) IgG
   4) IgE
   5) IgA

   a) Involved in allergic reactions
   b) A cell surface receptor with no known immunologic function
   c) Protects mucosal surfaces
   d) The first antibody produced during an immune response
   e) Crosses the placenta

6. Which of the following Ig subtypes can form multimers in serum?
   a) IgM
   b) IgG
   c) IgA
   d) IgM and IgG
   e) IgM and IgA

7. The specificity of antibody is determined by . . .
   a) the Fc domain.
   b) the variable region of the heavy chain.
   c) the flexibility of the hinge region.
   d) the three-dimensional structure formed by the variable region of both the light and heavy chain.
   e) the variable region of the light chain.

8. Match the process to its effect:
   1) Allelic exclusion
   2) Genetic recombination
   3) Alternative splicing
   4) Class switching
   5) Affinity maturation

   a) Changing surface bound antibody to secreted antibody
   b) ↑ antibody binding specificity during B-cell proliferation
   c) Each B-cell expresses antibody of one specificity
   d) The generation of antibody specificity
   e) Changing from IgM to IgG expression

9. Which of the following accurately describes the CD4 protein?
   a) CD4 is expressed on cytotoxic T cells, and binds to Class I MHC molecules
   b) CD4 is expressed on helper T cells, and binds to Class II MHC molecules
   c) CD4 is expressed on helper T cells, and binds to Class I MHC molecules
   d) CD4 is expressed on cytotoxic T cells, and binds to Class II MHC molecules
   e) CD4 is expressed on natural killer cells, and binds to Class I MHC molecules

10. Which of the following correctly describes the Th1/Th2 paradigm?
    a) Th1 cells secrete IL-4 and protect against parasites, whereas Th2 cells secrete IFN-γ and protect against intracellular infections
    b) Th1 cells secrete IFN-γ and protect against intracellular infections, whereas Th2 cells secrete IL-4 and protect against parasites
    c) Th1 cells secrete IL-4 and protect against intracellular infections, whereas Th2 cells secrete IFN-γ and protect against parasites
    d) Th1 cells secrete IFN-γ and protect against parasites, whereas Th2 cells secrete IL-4 and protect against intracellular infections
    e) Th1 cells secrete IL-4 and protect against parasites, whereas Th2 cells secrete IL-10 and protect against intracellular infections

11. Which of the following correctly describes Class I and Class II MHC molecules?
    a) Class I presents intracellular antigens to CD8 cells; Class II presents extracellular antigens to CD4 cells
    b) Class I presents extracellular antigens to CD8 cells; Class II presents intracellular antigens to CD4 cells
    c) Class I presents extracellular antigens to CD4 cells; Class II presents extracellular antigens to CD8 cells
    d) Both Class I and Class II present intracellular antigens to either CD4 or CD8 cells
    e) Neither Class I nor Class II is capable of presenting intracellular antigens

12. How are phagocytes recruited to the location of an infection?
    a) The brain sends out neurohormones to signal the location
    b) Phagocytes randomly leave the vasculature, and some happen to the area of infection by chance
    c) Phagocytes are summoned by chemotactic cytokines called chemokines, which are released by damaged cells and cells exposed to damaged host proteins
    d) Phagocytes are produced locally at the site of infection by proliferation of macrophages
    e) Phagocytes are recruited by antibodies

13. Match the following steps of extravasation to the cell-surface adhesins which mediate them:
    1) Rolling   a) PECAM
    2) Sticking   b) Selectins
    3) Diapedesis   c) ICAM

14. Which of the following statements is true?
    a) Innate immune cells possess memory and specificity
    b) Adaptive immune cells possess memory and specificity
    c) Innate immune cells possess memory, while adaptive immune cells possess specificity
    d) Innate immune cells possess specificity, while adaptive immune cells possess memory
    e) Both innate and adaptive immune cells possess memory and specificity

15. Which of the following statements regarding tolerance is true?
    a) Central tolerance is 100% effective
    b) Tolerance is mediated by antibodies
    c) Peripheral tolerance is strictly due to cryptic antigens
    d) Peripheral tolerance is an important back-up for central tolerance, which is imperfect
    e) Peripheral tolerance is strictly due to co-stimulation requirements

16. Match the following cytokines with their most important function:
    1) IL-1   a) Endogenous pyrogen
    2) IL-2   b) Immunosuppressive
    3) IL-4   c) Stimulates phagocytic activity/inflammation
    4) IL-10   d) T-cell activation
    5) IFN-γ e) Stimulates antibody production

17. Affinity maturation and class switching occur in which microanatomical site?
    a) Parafollicular areas of lymph nodes
    b) Bone marrow
    c) Mucosa
    d) Germinal centers in lymph node follicles
    e) Vascular compartment

18. Match the following types of immunodeficiencies with their key identifying characteristic:
    1) Primary B-cell deficiencies
    2) Primary T-cell deficiencies
    3) Phagocyte deficiencies
    4) Complement deficiencies
    5) Acquired B-cell deficiency

    a) Encapsulated bacterial infections starting in the teens
    b) Gingival dz, delayed umbilical cord separation, chronic abscesses
    c) Viral and bacterial infections starting as a neonate
    d) Encapsulated bacterial infections starting at 6 months
    e) Recurrent meningitis

19. Answer True or False to the following questions regarding AIDS:
    a) Homosexual transmission is the most common mode of HIV transmission worldwide.
    b) CD4 is sufficient for viral entry into T cells.
    c) HIV infection is 100% fatal without treatment.
    d) HIV is latent during the asymptomatic phase.
    e) The risk of opportunistic infections markedly increases when the CD4 count drops below 200.
    f) Homosexual HIV patients are more likely to develop Kaposi's Sarcoma.
    g) HIV patients can be effectively treated with two drugs.
    h) HIV can be cured in some people by highly active antiretroviral therapy (HAART).

20. A 34-year-old female presents to your emergency room complaining of tongue swelling, lip swelling, voice changes, and difficulty breathing. Just before you are about to intubate her to protect her airway she whispers to you that she has a complement deficiency. Which of the following is her most likely deficiency?
    a) C3 or C5 deficiency
    b) C2 or C4 deficiency
    c) C1 esterase deficiency
    d) C1 esterase inhibitor deficiency
    e) C6, C7, C8, or C9 deficiency

21. An 8-year-old male presents to your pediatric clinic with a long medical history of recurrent infections. Previous physicians have diagnosed him with Wiskott-Aldrich syndrome. What is the classic triad seen in these patients?
    a) High IgE levels, gargoyle facies, and recurrent bacterial infections
    b) Albinism, cranial neuropathies, and recurrent bacterial infections
    c) Eczema, thrombocytopenia, and recurrent bacterial infections
    d) Ataxia, telangiectasias, and recurrent respiratory infections

22. A 28-year-old male presents to your medical clinic with a complaint of recurrent sinus infections, chronic diarrhea, and asthma. He has been told that he has an immunodeficiency. Which of the following immunodeficiencies is most likely?
    a) Wiskott-Aldrich syndrome
    b) Severe combined immunodeficiency
    c) Chédiak-Higashi syndrome
    d) IgA deficiency
    e) Hyper IgM syndrome

23. A 7-month-old male status post a major heart operation presents with his mom to your pediatric clinic. He appears to have micrognathia and a short philtrum. Mother states that he has had episodes of tetany and multiple infections in the past necessitating hospital admission and intravenous medication treatment. Mom is tired of getting the run around regarding her son's medical condition and wants to know what is wrong with her son. Which of the following is the most likely cause of this child's symptoms?
    a) Common variable hypogammaglobulinemia
    b) Chédiak-Higashi syndrome
    c) Job's syndrome
    d) DiGeorge's syndrome
    e) Chronic granulomatous disease

24. Match the following types of hypersensitivity reactions with their identifying characteristic:

1) Allergic hypersensitivity	a) Serum sickness
2) Delayed type hypersensitivity	b) Anaphylaxis
3) Immune complex hypersensitivity	c) Erythroblastosis fetalis
4) Cytotoxic hypersensitivity	d) Poison ivy

25. Match the corresponding transplant reaction with its characteristic description:

1) Hyperacute graft rejection	a) Occurs within weeks of transplant
2) Acute graft rejection	b) Preformed antibodies in recipient's serum
3) Chronic graft rejection	c) Occurs months to years after transplant

ANSWERS

1. **d)** Antibody-dependent cell mediated cytotoxicity (ADCC) occurs when the constant region (Fc) of antibody binds to a phagocyte, and the non-specific phagocyte uses the variable portion of the antibody to provide specificity to recognize foreign microbes. This allows targeted digestion of the microbe, while sparing host tissues of the phagocyte's toxic molecules. In this instance, the antibody is only used by the phagocyte to recognize the microbe, and the antibody itself does not mediate any direct killing effect. ADCC is not used by lymphocytes, which are inherently specific due to their variable receptors.

2. **b)** Infections involving multicellular parasites (e.g., worms) typically cause eosinophilia if they are tissue invasive. Thus, organisms that are purely found in the gastrointestinal tract may not cause eosinophilia. *Trichinella*, the causative agent of trichinosis, widely invades parenchymal tissues, and causes a high grade eosinophilia. Neoplasms, particularly those involving white blood cells (leukemia and lymphoma), and any collagen-vascular disease leading to vasculitis also cause eosinophilia. For reasons that are not clear, *Coccidioides immitis* and *Aspergillus* fungal infections can cause eosinophilia, while eosinophilia is not typically seen in *Candida* infections.

3. **d)** Class II MHC (unlike Class I MHC, which is expressed on almost all nucleated cells) is only expressed on "professional antigen presenting cells." Professional antigen presenting cells are those that have two important properties: 1) they are phagocytic and 2) they express co-stimulatory molecules to activate T cells. Macrophages, B cells, and dendritic cells are the classical antigen presenting cells. Interestingly, when stimulated by interferon-γ, endothelial cells can present antigen via Class II MHC to T cells. T cells, on the other hand, do not present antigen to themselves, and are not antigen presenting cells.

4. **a)** An antibody is a tetramer, and can be thought of as a "dimer of dimers." Its subunit is one heavy chain bound to one light chain (a dimer), and two of these subunits comprise the final molecule (a dimer of the dimers).

5. **1-d, 2-b, 3-e, 4-a, 5-c.** Obviously the various Ig subclasses have multiple different functions, but those listed are the ones most important to remember for exams. IgM is always the first subclass produced. IgD has no known function other than as a surface receptor. IgG crosses the placenta, and is the mainstay of mature immune responses. IgE causes allergic reactions by cross-linking basophils and mast cells, and also is important in protection against worms. IgA is secreted across mucosal surfaces to protect them from external invaders.

6. **e)** IgM tends to form pentamers in serum, as the J chain connects 5 IgM molecules together by their Fc regions. IgA forms dimers by connection via a different J chain. IgG is always monomeric in serum.

7. **d)** The antigen-binding cleft is a three-dimensional surface comprising the intertwined variable regions of the light and heavy chains. The Fc region determines the subclass of Ig (e.g., IgM, IgD, IgG, etc.), but has nothing to do with antigen binding. The hinge region allows flexibility in the antibody, and also has nothing to do with antigen binding.

8. **1-c, 2-d, 3-a, 4-e, 5-b.** Allelic exclusion occurs when a B cell successfully rearranges a heavy chain and light chain allele, preventing any further rearrangements. This means the B cell can only express one type of heavy chain and light chain. Genetic recombination is the mechanism by which alleles are rearranged. Germ-line DNA is recombined to allow variable (V), diversity (D), and joining (J) gene segments to come together to form one V-D-J heavy chain allele, and V-J segments are combined to form one V-J light chain allele. Alternative splicing of messenger RNA can allow either inclusion or exclusion of the transmembrane domain of the coding region. Inclusion causes the mRNA to code for a surface bound protein while exclusion allows coding for a secreted protein. Class switching is the change from an IgM antibody of a given specificity to an IgG antibody of the same specificity. Affinity maturation is a natural selective process in which B cells expressing antibodies with higher affinities to the stimulating antigen are given survival signals. The result is that during an immune response, the affinity of generated antibody gets progressively higher.

9. **b)** The CD4 protein is a marker for helper T cells. It binds to Class II MHC molecules, thereby stabilizing the interaction between Class II MHC and the T cell receptor. The CD8 protein is a marker for cytotoxic T cells, and binds to Class I MHC molecules.

10. **b)** Th1 cells secrete high levels of IFN-γ, but do not secrete IL-4. IFN-γ stimulates phagocytic activity and inflammation, perfect for protection against intracellular pathogens. Th2 cells secrete high levels of IL-4, but do not secrete IFN-γ. IL-4 stimulates antibody production, and class switching to IgE, perfect for defense against parasites.

11. **a)** Intracellular, cytoplasmic antigens are pumped into the endoplasmic reticulum by the TAP complex, where such antigens bind to Class I MHC molecules. Class I MHC molecules present these cytoplasmic antigens to CD8 cells. Extracellular antigens, taken up by phagocytosis, bind to Class II MHC molecules in the phagolysosomes, and Class II MHC molecules present such antigens to CD4 cells.

12. **c)** Chemotactic cytokines, called chemokines, diffuse into the vascular compartment from their source in tissue exposed to trauma or infection. Such chemokines are secreted either by damaged cells themselves, or are secreted by neighboring cells alerted to the damage by exposure to host proteins leaked by the damaged cells. The chemokines set up a concentration gradient in the nearby vasculature, forming a sort of yellow-brick road that the phagocytes follow back to its source.

Antibodies and neurohormones are not directly involved in this recruitment. Macrophages are end-differentiated cells, and are not capable of cell division.

13. **1-b, 2-c, 3-a.** Rolling is caused by the loose binding of selectins on the endothelial cells to selectin receptors on the leukocyte. Sticking is due to a firmer attachment of ICAM on the endothelial cells to one of several ICAM receptors on the leukocyte. Diapedesis is the process by which the leukocyte squeezes in between neighboring endothelial cells, and binds to the molecule PECAM at the endothelial junction, using PECAM to pull itself across the endothelial monolayer.

14. **b)** Only adaptive immune cells (i.e., lymphocytes) possess memory and specificity. Innate immune cells (i.e., phagocytes) are non-specific and react to a given antigen in the same manner no matter how often they have been exposed to that antigen before. Memory allows lymphocytes to become more avid for a given antigen (affinity maturation), and to respond more quickly and with a more potent response with each successive exposure to the antigen.

15. **d)** Central tolerance involves deletion of auto-reactive T cells in the thymus. Since not all host antigens are expressed in the thymus, central tolerance cannot possibly tolerize T cells to all the different antigens in the host. Therefore, peripheral tolerance is an absolutely required fail-safe to prevent autoimmunity. Peripheral tolerance occurs outside of the thymus. Three main mechanisms cause peripheral tolerance. First, antigenic ignorance is the sequestration of host antigens from lymphocytes. If lymphocytes never see a given host antigen, none can ever become reactive to it. Second, recognition of antigen is not enough for a T cell to be turned on. Instead, the antigen-presenting cell must co-stimulate the T cell by expressing a second stimulating marker. Antigen-presenting cells only express these second signals when the antigen-presenting cells have been exposed to some danger signal in the environment (e.g., microbial fractions or inflammatory cytokines). Finally, we do not mount reactions to foodstuffs because TGF-β in the gut tolerizes T cells to gastrointestinal antigens (so-called oral tolerance).

16. **1-a, 2-d, 3-e, 4-b, 5-c.** IL-1 is synthesized by most human cell types and released upon damage to the cell (it is thus a danger signal). It directly stimulates the fever response in the hypothalamus. IL-2 is the *sine qua non* for T-cell proliferation; when you think IL-2, think T-cells. IL-4 is a key cytokine for stimulating antibody production; when you think IL-4, think antibodies. IL-10 is probably the most immunosuppressive cytokine known. It shuts down expression of almost every cytokine, including itself, and inhibits inflammation. IFN-γ is crucial to stimulating phagocytes to uptake and kill microbes.

17. **d)** The germinal centers of lymph node follicles are the sites of massive B-cell proliferation following activation by antigen. During this

proliferation, the lymphoblasts undergo a million-fold increase in the mutation rate only at the Ig loci (remarkably, the mutation rate does not increase elsewhere in the genome). The presence of antigen which continues to select for high affinity B-cell receptor binding, combined with an environment of rapid mutation, leads to Darwinian evolution of the B cells in the germinal center. Thus, only those B-cells whose Ig mutations lead to higher affinity binding are selected to continue to grow. The result is affinity maturation. Class switching also occurs here due to T cell help provided by CD40-ligand binding to CD40 on the B cells.

18. **1-d, 2-c, 3-b, 4-e, 5-a.** Phenotypes in patients with primary B-cell deficiencies do not appear until maternal IgG is cleared from the newborn child's serum. This process takes about six months, so with good clinical reliability (and 100% reliability on standardized exams), primary B-cell deficiencies present AT AGE 6 MONTHS! B-cell defects allow infections by encapsulated bacteria (e.g., *Hemophilus, Streptococcus, E. coli*, etc.). Conversely, T-cell deficiencies allow infections by both viruses and bacteria (as well as fungi), but these present within weeks of birth, allowing an easy time-course differentiation from B-cell defects. Phagocyte deficiencies allow a variety of infections but clinically the lack of phagocytes prevents easy separation of the umbilical cord (phagocytes chew off the cord by secreting lytic enzymes), allow terrible gingival disease to set in, and prevent the resolution of simple skin and subcutaneous infections, causing chronic abscesses. There are many different kinds of complement deficiencies; however, the most famous (and most testable) are deficiencies in components of the membrane attack complex (MAC). MAC is crucial to protection against *Neisseria*, so these patients get recurrent *N. meningitidis* meningitis. In fact, *N. meningitidis* is so susceptible to antibiotics that any patient who fails therapy and recrudesces should immediately be screened for complement deficiencies. Acquired B-cell defect refers to common variable hypogammaglobulinemia, a defect whose pathogenesis is not understood. This presents with encapsulated bacterial infections starting any time between the teen years to young adulthood.

19. a) **False**—heterosexual is most common worldwide

   b) **False**—along with CD4, a co-receptor such as CCR5 or CXCR4 are needed for viral entry

   c) **False**—about 5% of HIV infected patients are Long Term Nonprogressors, who never get sick for unclear reasons

   d) **False**—HIV has no latent phase in its life-cycle, the asymptomatic period is due to immune reconstitution keeping pace with HIV-mediated T-cell destruction

   e) **True**—this is why all patients with CD4 counts below 200 should be started on Bactrim prophylaxis

f) True—Kaposi's Sarcoma is due to co-infection with Human Herpes Virus 8, which is more commonly transmitted during homosexual sex, thus it is in fact important in a sick HIV patient to find out how he or she acquired the disease, because the differential diagnosis of opportunistic infections differs somewhat depending upon the route of HIV transmission

g) False—standard of care is three or more anti-retrovirals

h) False—although the virus can be suppressed below the limit of detectability in the majority of patients, there is NO EVIDENCE that these patients are cured, and indeed when investigators have stopped drug therapy after several years of total suppression, the virus has invariably repopulated itself from latent reservoirs in the lymph system. (Although some investigators think cure might be possible if suppression is maintained for long enough to allow memory T cells, which harbor the virus, to die—this might require 30 years or more of therapy!)

20. **d)** C1 esterase inhibitor is the cause of this patient's angioedema. C2 & C4 presents with a lupus like disorder, C3 or C5 present with recurrent bacterial infections. C6–9 deficiency affect the formation of the membrane attack complex and present with recurrent *Neisseria* infections.

21. **c)** Eczema, thrombocytopenia, and recurrent bacterial infections. The other choices correspond to a) Job's syndrome, b) Chédiak-Higashi, e) Ataxia-Telangiectasia.

22. **d)** Ig A deficiency. IgA is commonly found in respiratory secretions pt's classically present with sinusitis and respiratory complaints. a) See above. b) SCID children are sick within weeks of birth and are susceptible to everything. c) See above. e) CD 40 defect prevents IgG class switching.

23. **d)** DiGeorge's syndrome is an embryologic defect in pharyngeal pouch 3&4 causing parathyroid aplasia and thymic aplasia. Patients present with hypocalcemia and T-cell deficiency. Other choices: a) would present with bacterial infections onsetting at ages 15–35, with splenomegaly and lymphadenopathy; b) would present with albinism and neuropathy in addition to infections; c) would present with elevated IgE levels, gargoyle facies, etc.; e) would present with recurrent bacterial infections, typically skin/soft tissue infections or visceral abscesses (especially liver).

24. **1-b, 2-d, 3-a, 4-c**

25. **1-b, 2-a, 3-c**

Microbiology and Immunology Review Questions & Answers: A Self-Assessment Test

MICROBIOLOGY AND IMMUNOLOGY REVIEW: A SELF-ASSESSMENT TEST

QUESTIONS

A 4-year-old boy is brought to the emergency room by her parents for a high spiking fever, as well as abdominal pain, nausea, and vomiting. The fevers and pain have been getting worse for several days. The child has a history of several prior serious skin infections, each of which resolved with antibiotics. On exam, the boy is febrile to 102°F. He appears in moderate distress, and his belly is tender, particularly in the right upper quadrant. A CT scan of the abdomen reveals a liver abscess. Antibiotic therapy is initiated and a drainage procedure is performed. Gram stain of the drained pus reveals purple-stained cocci in cluster formations, and on culture the organism displays complete hemolysis of blood agar and coagulase activity. A suspicious pediatric infectious disease specialist orders testing that reveals a defect in the ability of the boy's white blood cells to produce oxidative radicals, such as O_2^-.

1. What organism cultured out of the boy's liver abscess?

   a) *Streptococcus pyogenes*

   b) *Streptococcus pneumonia*

   c) *Staphylococcus aureus*

   d) *Staphylococcus epidermidis*

   e) *Escherichia coli*

2. Based on the results of the lack of superoxide production by the child's white blood cells, he is diagnosed with a congenital immunodeficiency. Two years later the boy develops a life-threatening infection with a strange organism. Tissue histopathology of a biopsy of a skin lesion on the patient shows which of the following?

   a) Gram positive rods appearing like "box-cars in a train"

   b) Gram negative coccobacilli that exhibit bipolar staining

   c) Fungi with both hyphae and pseudohyphae

   d) A septate mold branching at 45°

   e) A nonseptate mold branching at 90°

3. A 23-year-old female recent immigrant from Mexico presents to the emergency room with new onset seizures. A CT scan of the brain reveals ring-enhancing lesions with significant edema. Also seen are small, calcific dots in other areas of the brain. Which of the following parasites is the most likely cause of her seizures?
   a) *Diphyllobothrium latum*
   b) *Echinococcus*
   c) *Taenia saginata*
   d) *Taenia solium*
   e) *Paragonimus*

4. An 18-year-old college student presents to the emergency room with headaches, fever, nausea, and vomiting. He has a stiff neck on exam, and his lumbar puncture confirms the diagnosis of meningitis. Which of the following organisms would not be a common cause of the patient's meningitis?
   a) *Streptococcus pneumonia*
   b) *Hemophilus influenza*
   c) *Neisseria meningitidis*
   d) *Listeria monocytogenes*
   e) *Pseudomonas aeruginosa*

5. The Gram stain from the same patient's cerebrospinal fluid shows gram negative diplococci. A defect of which of the following host defense mechanisms is most likely to be present?
   a) T cells
   b) B cells
   c) Complement
   d) Phagocytes
   e) Combined immunodeficiency

6. A 34-year-old male who returned from a trip to Mexico several days ago presents with abdominal pain, bloody diarrhea, and fever. Which of the following gram negative rods is an unlikely cause of his dysentery?
   a) *Enterobacter*
   b) *E. coli*
   c) *Salmonella*
   d) *Shigella*
   e) *Yersinia*

7. Each of the organisms listed in question 6 is a member of the Enterobacteriacea. Which of the following characteristics does not define membership in this group?
   a) Normal flora in the respiratory tract
   b) Ferment glucose
   c) Are facultative anaerobes
   d) Are oxidase negative
   e) Reduce nitrates to nitrites

8. A 40-year-old Filipino male who recently returned from a trip to Arizona presents to the hospital with fevers, headaches, and a skin lesion. Of note, an earthquake had occurred during the patient's stay in Arizona. He has been self-medicating with ibuprofen and amoxicillin. The patient is eosinophilic, with an absolute eosinophil count of 1500 per microliter in peripheral blood. His lumbar puncture reveals evidence of meningitis. Which of the following is not in the differential diagnosis of the patient's eosinophilia?
   a) Lymphoma
   b) Allergy to medications
   c) Systemic lupus erythematosus
   d) Fungal infections
   e) *Staphylococcus aureus*

9. What is the most likely cause of this patient's meningitis?
   a) *Aspergillus*
   b) *Coccidioides immitis*
   c) *Enterobacter*
   d) *Histoplasma capsulatum*
   e) *Clonorchis sinensis*

10. Match the following terms with their descriptions:

    1) Allelic exclusion
    2) Affinity maturation
    3) Class switching
    4) Fab domain
    5) Mitogen

    a) Responsible for choosing the type of Fc produced
    b) Type 1 T-cell independent antigen
    c) No two antibody or T-cell receptors are made by the same lymphocyte
    d) The antigen binding portion
    e) IgG binds to antigen more avidly than IgM

11. Which of the following is not true of HIV infection?
    a) Patients with CD4 T-cell counts less than 500 per microliter should take trimethoprim-sulfamethoxazole prophylaxis
    b) Patients should never receive less than 3 drug antiretroviral therapy
    c) Worldwide, homosexual contact is not the most common mode of transmission
    d) HIV enters cells by binding to CD4 and either CCR5 or CXCR4
    e) At least 95% of patients infected with HIV will die from opportunistic infections or other AIDS-associated diseases without antiretroviral therapy

12. Which of the following mechanisms may predispose people to autoimmunity?
    a) Central tolerance
    b) Antigenic ignorance
    c) Co-stimulation
    d) Oral tolerance
    e) Type 1 immunity

13. A 6-month-old female is brought to the emergency room for fevers and vomiting. The infant's lumbar puncture is positive, revealing gram positive cocci in chains on Gram stain. The culture grows an organism that causes synergistic hemolysis with a lab strain of S. aureus. The patient had been healthy until 6 months of age, but in subsequent months, the child develops recurrent respiratory and intestinal infections, often caused by S. pneumonia and H. influenza. The patient has normal numbers of peripheral B cells. What organism caused the patient's initial episode of meningitis at the age of 6 months?
    a) S. pneumonia
    b) S. pyogenes
    c) Enterococcus
    d) S. agalactiae
    e) E. coli

14. The patient from question 13 most likely has which of the following immunodeficiencies?
    a) Bruton's agammaglobulinemia
    b) Selective IgA/IgG deficiency
    c) DiGeorge's syndrome
    d) Wiskott-Aldrich syndrome
    e) Chédiak-Higashi syndrome

15. A 50-year-old male with a history of intravenous drug use presents to the hospital with fevers, weight loss, malaise, and new skin lesions over the last several weeks. On exam, the patient is febrile to 102°C. He has poor dentition, conjunctival petechiae, an impressive aortic murmur, splenomegaly, and a tender nodule on his thumb. A diagnosis of endocarditis is confirmed by echocardiography. A blood culture grows gram positive cocci. Which of the following is an unlikely cause of the patient's endocarditis?

    a) Viridans group *Streptococcus*

    b) *Staphylococcus*

    c) *Enterococcus*

    d) *Mycobacterium tuberculosis*

    e) *Streptococcus bovis*

16. The gram positive cocci mentioned in question 15 are γ-hemolytic, resist bile, hydrolyze esculin, and are inhibited by hypertonic saline. Which of the following tests must now be done for the patient?

    a) Test the organism for vancomycin-susceptibility

    b) Colonoscopy

    c) Coagulase test of the organism

    d) Quellung test of the organism

    e) Novobiocin test of the organism

17. Match the following term with the appropriate organism.

1) Spelunking	a) *Listeria*
2) Broad-based bud	b) *Mucor*
3) Tumbling motility	c) *Vibrio*
4) Diabetic ketoacidosis	d) *Histoplasma*
5) "Rice-water" stool	e) *Blastomyces*

18. A 20-year-old presents with jaundice, malaise, fevers, weight loss, and lymphadenopathy. Laboratories reveal elevated transaminase levels. Which of the following viruses is not likely a cause of the hepatitis?

    a) CMV

    b) Hepatitis A virus

    c) Hepatitis B virus

    d) Adenovirus

    e) EBV

19. The same patient from question 18 is diagnosed with mononucleosis. However, his heterophile antibody is negative. Which of the following can cause heterophile-negative mononucleosis, along with CMV?
    a) *Pseudomonas*
    b) JC Polyomavirus
    c) BK Polyomavirus
    d) HTLV
    e) *Toxoplasma gondii*

20. Match the following zoonoses with their exposure/syndrome (use each answer only once):

    1) A bat flies into a rural cabin where people are sleeping
    2) Cleaning up mice droppings in a Southwestern desert
    3) People swimming in a lake develop meningitis and renal failure
    4) Drinking milk straight from a cow
    5) Helping a cow to give birth on a farm

    a) *Coxiella*
    b) *Leptospira*
    c) Rabies
    d) *Brucella*
    e) Hantavirus

21. Match the following cell type with their receptor or characteristic:

    1) T-helper cell
    2) T-cytotoxic cell
    3) NK cell
    4) Th2 cell
    5) γδ T cell

    a) Activity inhibited by MHC I
    b) Binds to antigen + MHC II
    c) Expresses CD8
    d) Expresses IL-4
    e) Does not require antigen processing

22. A 22-year-old male presents to an outpatient clinic for routine follow up of his recent diagnosis of genital herpes, which had been made by another physician based on the exam finding of a non-tender penile ulcer. Being an astute clinician, you realize that the patient may have been misdiagnosed, as herpes-associated ulcers are typically painful. On your exam, you discover a diffuse maculopapular rash, including on the patient's palms and soles. The remainder of the exam is normal. Which of the following tests will confirm the diagnosis?
    a) Allergy testing to the acyclovir the patient was given for his herpes
    b) *Rickettsia* serologies
    c) Biopsy for vasculitis
    d) RPR
    e) Echocardiography and blood cultures

23. What other test should the patient in question 22 receive while he is in clinic with you?
    a) Heterophile antibody
    b) Culture of the maculopapular lesions
    c) HIV test
    d) Quantitative immunoglobulins
    e) Urine toxicology screen

24. Match the clinical syndrome with the type of hypersensitivity reaction:
    1) Type 1   a) Serum sickness
    2) Type 2   b) PPD test
    3) Type 3   c) Penicillin-related anaphylaxis
    4) Type 4   d) Penicillin-related hemolytic anemia

25. An otherwise healthy 26-year-old medical student comes to Employee Health for a routine evaluation. His PPD is 12 mm. Which of the following is true/correct?
    a) The PPD is positive
    b) The student's PPD is only positive if he/she is also HIV positive
    c) Appropriate treatment for latent TB requires 6 months of therapy, unless he/she is HIV positive, in which case 9 months are required
    d) The student's PPD is positive unless he/she has been BCG vaccinated, in which case the PPD is unreliable
    e) If the student was 40 years old, he/she should not receive INH therapy

26. Questions 26–30 refer to a 44-year-old otherwise healthy male who traveled to a rural area in the southeast for vacation. While there he participated in numerous outdoor activities, including hiking. He then developed a febrile, flu-like illness and went to the hospital for evaluation. He was leukopenic and thrombocytopenic, and the laboratory technician noted intracellular inclusion bodies within the patient's neutrophils. The patient also had elevated transaminase levels. What is the most likely causative organism of this patient's febrile illness?
    a) Dengue virus
    b) *Rickettsia*
    c) *Anaplasma*
    d) *Babesia*
    e) *Plasmodium*

27. Suppose the same patient had instead traveled to Martha's Vineyard, and had had a splenectomy as a young man. He presented with a flu-like illness, and instead of leukopenia and thrombocytopenia, and he had a severe hemolytic anemia, with rapidly worsening hemo-dynamic status. The intracellular inclusion bodies were seen in the patient's red cells, rather than his leukocytes. Now what is the most likely diagnosis?

    a) Dengue virus
    b) *Rickettsia*
    c) *Ehrlichia*
    d) *Babesia*
    e) *Plasmodium*

28. Now suppose the same patient from question 26 instead presented with a rapidly progressing rash, consisting of diffuse petechia starting on the palms and soles and progressing inwards to the trunk. The patient is in disseminated intravascular coagulation, and his hemodynamics are compromised. Now what is the most likely diagnosis?

    a) Dengue virus
    b) *Rickettsia*
    c) *Ehrlichia*
    d) *Babesia*
    e) *Plasmodium*

29. The same patient from question 26 has instead traveled to Costa Rica and spent time traipsing through the rain forest. Ten days later he develops a severe headache, high spiking fever, and diffuse myalgias. The patient is febrile to 104°C and complains that his body aches are so severe that he feels like his bones are breaking. He has no rash, but is slightly leukopenic and thrombocytopenic, and has transaminitis. He has been taking doxycycline. Now what is the most likely diagnosis?

    a) Dengue virus
    b) *Rickettsia*
    c) *Ehrlichia*
    d) *Babesia*
    e) *Plasmodium*

30. Finally, the same patient from question 26, having traveled to Costa Rica and spent time in the rain forest, presents with high spiking fever, myalgias, and the same lab abnormalities. However the patient was instead taking chloroquine prophylaxis and he stopped it a week after getting back home. Intracellular forms are seen in the patient's red blood cells. Now what is the most likely diagnosis?
    a) Dengue virus
    b) *Rickettsia*
    c) *Ehrlichia*
    d) *Babesia*
    e) *Plasmodium*

31. Patients infected with HIV are at higher risk than the general population for each of the following diseases, except:
    a) Tuberculosis
    b) Syphilis
    c) *Streptococcus pneumonia*
    d) Lymphoma
    e) Colon cancer

32. A 20-year-old African American male with sickle cell anemia presents to the hospital with worsening fatigue and pallor. His hemoglobin is 4 mg/dL but there is no evidence of sickling on the peripheral blood smear. The patient's reticulocyte count is very low. His mother recently had a febrile illness that then developed into a diffuse polyarticular arthritis in her. What is the most likely etiology?
    a) Adenovirus
    b) Molluscum contagiosum
    c) HSV-1
    d) VZV
    e) Parvovirus B19

33. A 20-year-old patient is referred to you because of an abnormal lab. The patient has a history of recurrent skin infections, presenting with strangely non-inflammatory skin boils, without significant erythema or heat, and they typically grow *S. aureus.* The patient has also had recurrent pneumonias, and has developed blebs on chest x-ray. He has a syndromic facies, with a prominent brow and fleshy nose. His dental x-rays reveal strange, double-rows of teeth. What is the most likely lab abnormality that brought this patient to your office?
    a) WBC count of 50,000/μL
    b) Elevated IgE levels
    c) Lack of B cells
    d) Lack of T cells
    e) Abnormally shaped neutrophils

34. A 45-year-old business man goes on a bear-hunting trip. Having successfully killed his bear, the man decides it would be a good idea to prove his virility by opening the bear up and drinking its bile (don't laugh, this case really happened, and is a well-known phenomenon). Two weeks later he presents to the hospital with the bear's posthumous revenge, with fevers to 104°C, periorbital edema, severe myalgias, elevated muscle enzymes, and an eosinophil count of 50,000/µL. What is the diagnosis?
    a) *Strongyloides*
    b) *Dracunculus*
    c) *Trichinella*
    d) *Onchocerca*
    e) *Ascaris*

35. Each of the following are characteristics of congenital syphilis except:
    a) Chancre
    b) Saber shins
    c) "Snuffles"
    d) Hutchinson's teeth
    e) Saddle nose

36. Group A *Streptococcus* is responsible for each of the following diseases, except:
    a) Necrotizing fasciitis
    b) Post-infectious glomerulonephritis
    c) Rheumatic fever
    d) Scarlet fever
    e) Cholecystitis

37. Rheumatic fever is caused by a result of what immunologic process?
    a) Antibody-dependent cell mediated cytotoxicity (ADCC)
    b) Molecular mimicry
    c) Angioedema
    d) Anergy
    e) Hybridoma

38. Match the vector with the disease it carries:
    1) *Anopheles* mosquito   a) *Borrelia*
    2) Reduviid bug   b) *Trypanosoma gambiense*
    3) Tsetse fly   c) *Leishmania*
    4) Sandfly   d) *Plasmodium*
    5) *Ixodes*   e) *Trypanosoma cruzi*

39. The following serotypes of HPV are known causes of cervical cancer except:
    a) 16
    b) 18
    c) 31
    d) 33
    e) 40

40. A 40-year-old healthy male presents to your office complaining of a growth on the back of his hand. The growth has been increasing in size for several weeks. The patient works in a tropical fish store and frequently cleans the tanks. A biopsy reveals granulomas with AFB organisms. What is the most likely causative organism?
    a) *Mycobacterium tuberculosis*
    b) *Mycobacterium marinum*
    c) *Mycobacterium leprum*
    d) *Nocardia*
    e) *Sporothrix schenckii*

41. A 56-year-old male presents to the hospital with flank pain and decreasing urinary output. A CT scan reveals that the patient has partial obstruction of the right kidney (hydroureter) caused by a massive kidney stone. The pH of the urine is 8.0. Gram negative rods are seen on Gram stain of the urine. What type of stone is most likely present?
    a) Calcium stone
    b) Uric acid stone
    c) Ammonium magnesium phosphate stone
    d) Marble

42. Match the antibody subtype with its key characteristic:
    1) IgM   a) Allergic reactions
    2) IgG   b) Mucosal secretions
    3) IgE   c) Crosses the placenta
    4) IgA   d) Polymerizes into pentamers

43. Match the cytokine with its key characteristic:
    1) IL-1   a) Stimulates eosinophil production
    2) IL-2   b) Stimulates fever
    3) IL-4   c) Stimulates T-cell proliferation
    4) IL-5   d) The key regulator of cell-mediated immunity
    5) IFN-γ (e) Stimulates B-cell activation/antibody production

44. A 60-year-old male smoker presented to the emergency room complaining of fever and productive cough. His chest x-ray revealed a lower lobar pneumonia. On further questioning, the patient indicated that he had severe diarrhea. His laboratories were significant for marked hyponatremia and a very high LDH. Despite his fever, his heart rate was only 60. What pathogen is most suggested by these findings?
    a) *Streptococcus pyogenes*
    b) *Mycoplasma*
    c) *Staphylococcus aureus*
    d) *Legionella*
    e) *M. tuberculosis*

45. What type of media must be used to grow the pathogen causing the pneumonia in question 44?
    a) Thayer Martin agar
    b) Maconkey agar
    c) Agar with Factor V (NAD) and Factor X (heme)
    d) Agar with iron and cysteine supplementation
    e) Bordet-Gengou agar

46. A 22-year-old diabetic female went swimming. Two days later she developed an infection in her ear. Over three days, the infection spread to the outside of her ear. She presents to the hospital with a bulging pinna and extreme tenderness on palpation. Examination reveals a severe otitis externa. What is the most likely cause of the infection?
    a) *Streptococcus pneumonia*
    b) *Pseudomonas*
    c) Coxsackie virus
    d) *Moraxella*
    e) *Hemophilus*

47. Match the virus with the characteristic disease it can cause:
1) Varicella virus	a) Tracheobronchitis
2) Coxsackie virus	b) Herpangina
3) Norwalk virus	c) Cruise ship diarrhea
4) Parainfluenza virus	d) Kaposi's sarcoma
5) Human Herpes Virus 8	e) Dermatomal pain

48. A 34-year-old male with a history of HIV presents to the emergency room with dyspnea on exertion, fevers, chills, weight loss, and a headache. He is hypoxic and is put on supplemental oxygen. His serum LDH is extremely high. His chest x-ray shows diffuse bilateral interstitial changes. His CD4 count is known to be less than 50 cells/μL. He is not on antiretroviral therapy, and is non-compliant with his antibiotic prophylaxis. His bacterial work up was negative. Bronchial lavage revealed the diagnosis. Which of the following is the most likely diagnosis?

    a) CMV
    b) *Pneumocystis*
    c) Lymphoma
    d) Kaposi's sarcoma
    e) *Aspergillus*

49. The same patient from question 48 is being treated for his pneumonia. However, the patient's headache continues to worsen. A lumbar puncture is performed, revealing an opening pressure of 56 mm of water (<20 normal). The India ink test is positive. What is the diagnosis?

    a) *Coccidioides*
    b) *Histoplasma*
    c) *Cryptococcus*
    d) *Blastomyces*
    e) *Candida*

50. For the patient in question 48, you need to decide what prophylaxis to begin to prevent opportunistic infections. Which of the following regimens are appropriate?

    a) Levofloxacin
    b) Trimethoprim-sulfamethoxazole
    c) Azithromycin
    d) Trimethoprim-sulfamethoxazole + azithromycin
    e) Chloroquine

ANSWERS

1. **c)** *Staphylococcus aureus.* The culture grew a gram positive (purple staining) cocci in clusters. On the Boards (and on the wards also), anytime you see gram positive cocci in clusters, it is *Staphylococcus. Streptococcus,* conversely, is described as gram positive cocci in chains (or pairs for *S. pneumonia*). Furthermore, the organism exhibits complete hemolysis. *Staphylococcus* can do this, as can *S. pyogenes,* which is Group A β-hemolytic *Streptococcus.* Remember that β-hemolysis means complete hemolysis. In contrast, *S. pneumonia* exhibits α, or incomplete, hemolysis. The coagulase test is used to distinguish *S. aureus* (coagulase positive) from *S. epidermidis* (coagulase negative). *E. coli* is a gram negative rod.

2. **d) A septate mold branching at 45°.** This child has developed a lot of serious infections at a young age. The lack of superoxide production by his white blood cells is indicative of chronic granulomatous disease (CGD). Patients with CGD are at risk for infections caused by catalase + organisms, such as *S. aureus* and *Aspergillus. Aspergillus* is septate and branches at 45°, in contrast to the molds that cause *Mucor,* which are nonseptate and branch at 90°. Gram positive rods that appear like box-cars in a train refers to *Bacillus* species, gram negative coccobacilli that exhibit bipolar staining refers to *Yersinia,* and only fungus that grows as pseudohyphae is *Candida.* It is *S. aureus* and *Aspergillus,* however, that are much more commonly seen in patients with CGD.

3. **d)** *Taenia solium.* The patient has neurocysticercosis. New onset seizures in a Latin American immigrant are due to neurocysticercosis until proven otherwise. *Diphyllobothrium* is an intestinal tapeworm that causes weight loss and vitamin B_{12} deficiency. *Echinococcus* causes cysts, typically in the liver, that can result in anaphylaxis when they rupture. *Taenia saginata* is a beef tapeworm that causes minimal symptoms. *Paragonimus* is a lung fluke that causes hemoptysis.

4. **e)** *Pseudomonas aeruginosa.* Patients that are not in hospitals will rarely contract *Pseudomonas,* and *Pseudomonas* is not a cause of community acquired bacterial meningitis. Each of the other pathogens are well known to cause community acquired bacterial meningitis.

5. **c) Complement.** Although patients with invasive *Neisseria meningitidis* (gram negative diplococci) do not have to have any immunodeficiency, patients with defects in the late components of the complement cascade are at markedly increased risk for such infections. Defects in none of the other host defense mechanisms are associated with *Neisseria* infections.

6. **a)** *Enterobacter.* Unlike the other organisms, *Enterobacter* does not cause dysentery syndromes. Rather, it causes nosocomial infections

associated with lines, catheters, etc. Remember that *Yersinia entero-colitica* and *pseudotuberculosis* can cause dysentery (in contrast to *Y. pestis*, the cause of the bubonic plague).

7. **a) Normal flora in the respiratory tract.** The Enterobacteriacea are normal flora in the colon, not the respiratory tract. Each of the other characteristics defines membership in the family of the Enterobacteriacea.

8. **e) *Staphylococcus aureus*.** The purpose of this question is to alert you to disease states that present as eosinophilia. Remember the NAACP mnemonic: Neoplasm (often lymphoma), Allergy, *Aspergillus*/Addison's disease, *Coccidioides immitis*/Collagen Vascular disease (i.e., lupus), and Parasites. Pyogenic bacteria, such as *S. aureus*, do not cause eosinophilia.

9. **b) *Coccidioides immitis*.** There are several clues to this patient's diagnosis. First, a Filipino patient on the Boards has coccidioidomycosis until proven otherwise. For unclear reasons, Filipino and African American patients are at much higher risk for dissemination of coccidioidomycosis than are other patients. Second, the patient has been in the southwestern U.S. (Arizona). Third, earthquakes have been linked to outbreaks of coccidioidomycosis, likely because they kick dust up into the air, allowing the spores of the fungus to move around and get inhaled. *Aspergillus* is a very uncommon cause of meningitis, as is *Enterobacter*. *Histoplasma* would be acquired in the Midwestern river valleys, not in Arizona. *Clonorchis* does not cause meningitis; it causes biliary tract obstruction and is associated with cholangiocarcinoma.

10. **1-c, 2-e, 3-a, 4-d, 5-b.** Allelic exclusion is a genetic even that shuts down production of the alternate, as of yet unexpressed allele of T- or B-cell receptor genes, thereby limiting lymphocytes to making T-cell receptors or antibody (i.e., B-cell receptors) of one specificity only. Affinity maturation is the phenomenon whereby natural selection in the lymph node follicle acts to select only those B cells expressing highly avid antibody to continue to survive. Because affinity maturation occurs simultaneously with class switching, higher affinity antibodies are selected during the switch from IgM to IgG, and thus IgG antibody binds to antigen more avidly than does IgM. Class switching is the act by the B cell of swapping the constant portion (Fc) of IgM over to IgG, and then to IgA or IgE. The Fab domain of an antibody is the portion that actually binds to an antigen. Mitogens bypass the need for antigenic stimulation of B-cell proliferation; they are Type 1 T cell-independent antigens. In contrast, Type 2 T-cell independent antigens are large, complex structures with repeating domains that simply bind so strongly to B-cell antigen receptors that there is no need for a second signal from T cells.

11. **a)** Patients with CD4 T-cell counts less than 500 per µL should not take trimethoprim-sulfamethoxazole prophylaxis. Actually, the risk of

infection goes up when the CD4 count falls below 200 cells per μL, and this is the point at which prophylaxis is begun. All other statements are correct about HIV.

12. **e) Type 1 immunity.** Type 1 immunity is characterized by high levels of IFN-γ expression, resulting in powerful cell-mediated immunity and inflammation. Out of control Type 1 immunity has been linked to autoimmunity. Central and peripheral tolerance are mechanisms by which the immune system prevents autoimmunity. Antigenic ignorance, co-stimulation of lymphocytes, and oral tolerance are each subtypes of peripheral tolerance.

13. **d) *S. agalactiae*.** Group B Strep (*S. agalactiae*) is a common cause of meningitis in neonates and infants. A characteristic biochemical test identifying Group B Strep is CAMP factor positivity. CAMP factor synergizes with *S. aureus* to cause complete hemolysis. No other *Streptococcus* or *Enterococcus* species displays this biochemical feature. *E. coli* is not a gram positive cocci.

14. **b) Selective IgA/IgG deficiency.** The onset of infections at 6 months of age is a hallmark of antibody-deficiency syndromes, because this is the age at which maternal antibodies are cleared from the infant's blood, leaving the infant without antibody-mediated protection. Another hallmark of antibody deficiency diseases is the predominance of encapsulated bacteria, such as *S. pneumonia* and *H. influenza*, as a cause of the infections. Bruton's agammaglobulinemia is X-linked, and is therefore almost exclusively seen in boys. Also, B-cell numbers are not normal in this disease. In contrast, B-cell numbers are normal in selective IgA/IgG deficiency, in which the defect is class switching of antibody. DiGeorge's syndrome is a T-cell deficiency, in which infections are seen early after birth, and are accompanied by hypocalcemia and syndromic facies. Wiskott-Aldrich syndrome is also X-linked, and is typified by the triad of eczema, bacterial infections, and thrombocytopenia in boys. Chédiak-Higashi syndrome is a defect of phagocytes, and clinically presents with albinism and peripheral neuropathies, along with pyogenic bacterial infections.

15. **d) *Mycobacterium tuberculosis*.** Endocarditis is a very uncommon manifestation of TB, and *M. tuberculosis* is not a gram positive cocci. Viridans *Streptococci* cause endocarditis from gingival sources. The patient's drug use is a risk for *Staphylococcus*, and *Enterococcus* and *S. bovis* cause bacteremia/endocarditis from gut sources.

16. **b) Colonoscopy.** Group D Strep (*S. bovis*) is γ-hemolytic, resistant to bile, hydrolyzes esculin, and is inhibited by hypertonic saline. Bacteremia caused by Group D Strep is strongly associated with the presence of colonic tumor or malignancy, and this must be ruled out in this patient. Vancomycin susceptibility would be an issue for *Enterococcus*, which is increasingly resistant (VRE). Coagulase and novobiocin are tests done for *Staphylococcus*. Quellung test confirms

the presence of a capsule on a bacteria, and is most often used to identify *S. pneumonia.*

17. **1-d, 2-e, 3-a, 4-b, 5-c.** If a patient goes spelunking in the Midwest, particularly in a cave filled with bats and near a river bank, they are infected with Histoplasmosis until proven otherwise on a Board exam. Broad-based bud is the description of *Blastomyces* in a tissue section on the Boards. Tumbling motility is characteristic of *Listeria.* Every patient in diabetic ketoacidosis who has any eye, face, or head complaint has mucormycosis until proven otherwise on the Boards. "Rice-water" stool is the classic description of the diarrhea seen in patients with cholera.

18. **d) Adenovirus.** Adenovirus is a common cause of upper respiratory infections, and can also cause pharyngoconjunctival fever, which presents with conjunctivitis and pharyngitis. Transaminitis is common during mononucleosis, caused either by CMV or EBV, and of course occurs during acute Hepatitis A and B infection.

19. **e) *Toxoplasma gondii.*** *T. gondii* is the third most common cause of mononucleosis, behind EBV and CMV. *Pseudomonas* causes nosocomial infections in sick, hospitalized patients, not mononucleosis. JC Polyomavirus is the cause of Progressive Multifocal Leukoencephalopathy in AIDS patients. BK Polyomavirus causes renal transplant rejection. HTLV causes tropical spastic paraparesis, and is associated with T-cell leukemia.

20. **1-c, 2-e, 3-b, 4-d, 5-a.** In the U.S., rabies is most commonly caused by exposures to bats, and in some cases no direct bite has been reported. Thus, on the Boards, if a bat flies into a patient's room, even if no bite occurs, prophylax for rabies! Hantavirus cases have occurred in people living in rural cabins in the southwestern deserts, where lots of mice droppings are found. Leptospirosis occurs in people who swim in fresh or saltwater where animals urinate. *Brucella* is most commonly associated with unpasteurized milk intake. Farm animal birth products or placenta are a classically rich source of *Coxiella.*

21. **1-b, 2-c, 3-a, 4-d, 5-e.** T-helper cells are CD4+ T lymphocytes that bind to antigen in the context of MHC II. T-cytotoxic cells are CD8+ T lymphocytes that bind to antigen in the context of MHC I. NK cells do not kill host cells that express MHC I. Th2 cells are CD4+ T lymphocytes that express IL-4 and do not express IFN-γ. $\gamma\delta$ T cells can bind directly to antigens by their T-cell receptors, and do not require that antigen be processed and presented in the context of MHC molecules.

22. **d) RPR.** A painless penile ulcer that self-heals is typical of a chancre, and the maculopapular rash involving the palms and soles are classic for secondary syphilis. The RPR is virtually 100% sensitive in this setting. Acyclovir allergy does not commonly cause a rash. There is no reason

to believe the patient has either *Rickettsia* or vasculitis, nor is there evidence for endocarditis.

23. **c) HIV test.** Everyone with a sexually transmitted disease should have an HIV test! All the other answers are irrelevant to this case. Heterophile antibodies are used to detect EBV associated mononucleosis. *T. pallidum* cannot be cultured. Quantitative immunoglobulins are used to work up immunodeficiencies, and there is no indication for a urine toxicology screen on this patient.

24. **1-c, 2-d, 3-a, 4-b.** Type 1 hypersensitivity reactions are caused by pre-sensitized IgE-mediated activation of mast cells, and cause clinical anaphylaxis. Type 2 reactions are caused by direct antibody-mediated binding to hapten conjugates, such as penicillin-breakdown products binding to red cells or platelets. This can result in antibody-mediated destruction of red cells or platelets. Type 3 reactions are caused by complement activation mediated by immune complexes of antibody and antigen, such as are seen in serum sickness. Type 4 is the classic delayed type hypersensitivity reaction, utilized so effectively in the PPD test.

25. **a) The PPD is positive.** Because the medical student works in a health care setting, 10 mm is the appropriate cut-off for positivity. PPDs in HIV patients are positive if the PPD is ≥5 mm. The duration of treatment for latent TB is 9 months for all patients, regardless of HIV status. BCG vaccination is not taken into account when interpreting PPDs. The exposure history to BCG is ignored. Since 2000, the guidelines have specifically stated that everyone with a positive PPD should receive treatment for latent infection (assuming active disease is ruled out); age is no longer a contraindication to treatment for latent infection.

26. **c) *Anaplasma* (formerly *Ehrlichia*).** On the Boards, leukopenia, thrombocytopenia, and transaminitis should immediately suggest *Anaplasma phagocytophila* or *Ehrlichia chaffeensis*, particularly in a hiker, or someone exposed to ticks. These infections are typically acquired in the southeast. The finding of intracellular inclusion bodies within neutrophils also strongly suggests the diagnosis. Dengue would be expected in a traveler to a foreign country, especially Latin America or other tropical area, and would not cause intracellular inclusions. *Rickettsia* are also acquired by ticks, and can also cause leukopenia and thrombocytopenia, however rashes are typically present. *Babesia* is suggested by an intracellular ring-lesion within red blood not cells, neutrophils, and is often accompanied by hemolytic anemia. *Plasmodium* would be acquired in foreign, tropical countries.

27. **d) *Babesia*.** First of all, if Martha's Vineyard is on the Boards, the answer is *Babesia* until proven otherwise. It is typically transmitted via tick bite in the New England area, specifically along the coast. As well, splenectomy is a major risk factor for a severe hemolytic anemia in patients with *Babesia* infections. The intracellular inclusions in red

blood cells are another key feature of *Babesia* infections. Keep in mind that *Babesia* and *Ehrlichia* are common co-infectants, and occasionally *Rickettsia* as well. So testing/treating for all of them is reasonable.

28. **b)** *Rickettsia.* The key is the rash. Although *Anaplasma, Ehrlichia, Babesia,* and *Rickettsia* all cause febrile, flu-like illnesses, with myalgias and abdominal pain, and all are acquired by tick bites in the same general area of the U.S. (east/southeast), only *Rickettsia* is commonly associated with a rash. Note that one would not see inclusion bodies in red or white cells with *Rickettsia* infections.

29. **a) Dengue virus.** So now we have a patient having traveled to Latin America, and particularly a tropical part of Latin America, with significant mosquito exposure (in the rain forest). Thousands of cases of Dengue occur in this part of the world every year. The very high fever, lack of rash, and the same lab abnormalities seen in patients with *Ehrlichia* are typical. Patients complaining of particularly severe myalgias or bone pain, possibly even describing the sensation as feeling as if the bones are breaking, are key buzzwords for Dengue on the Boards. Although malaria can cause all of these same findings in the same patient (i.e., mosquito exposure, tropical country), the myalgias/bone pain will not be as strongly emphasized on the Boards, and use of doxycycline or another malarial prophylaxis strategy make malaria less likely.

30. **e)** *Plasmodium.* Malaria an extremely common infection to be acquired in travelers. The point of this series of questions has been to emphasize the overlap of the common signs, symptoms, and laboratory findings of the listed diseases. Key buzzwords will help you distinguish amongst them, as will location of travel. For malaria, lack of prophylaxis, or on the Boards, even more important, incomplete prophylaxis, should make you immediately suspect malaria. Remember that *Plasmodium vivax/ovale* have latent forms in the liver, and can relapse weeks to months (or in rare cases, years) after acquisition of infection if prophylaxis was not taken for the appropriate period after coming home (usually requires 4 weeks of continued prophylaxis upon return). Also, malaria and *Babesia* present with red cell inclusions; the other diseases do not.

31. **e) Colon cancer.** HIV patients have much higher risks of developing each of the other diseases, as well as *Mycobacterium avium intracellulare* (MAI), *Toxoplasma* encephalitis, CMV retinitis/colitis, *Cryptococcus, Histoplasma,* etc. The risk is directly related to CD4 counts, antibiotic prophylaxis should be started in these patients to prevent many of these opportunistic infections.

32. **e) Parvovirus B19.** This is a classic presentation of parvovirus-induced aplastic anemia, which causes a profoundly severe anemia in patients with underlying blood dyscrasias. The anemias are not hemolytic; they are hypoproliferative due to targeting of the virus to red cell precursors in the bone marrow. In healthy adults parvovirus B19

causes a flu-like illness followed by arthritis. In children it causes Fifth Disease, or slapped cheek disease, a benign infection that causes erythema on the cheeks and a mild fever. In fetuses it can be fatal, causing hydrops fetalis.

33. **b) Elevated IgE levels.** The patient has Job's Syndrome. The recurrent pulmonary infections, resulting in blebs, recurrent "cold abscesses" caused by *S. aureus*, classic gargoyle facies, and pathognomonic double-rows of teeth on dental x-rays, are typical. The other lab abnormalities are not associated with these findings.

34. **c) *Trichinella*.** This is all typical of trichinosis. It is acquired by eating undercooked pork or game meat (including polar bear, brown bear, walrus, etc.). Periorbital edema, severe myalgia with elevated muscle enzymes, and extremely high eosinophil counts are features seen in trichinosis. *Strongyloides* can cause eosinophilia, but the muscle findings and periorbital edema would be atypical. *Dracunculus* is a rare infection found only in Africa, in which large worms extrude out of the skin, typically in the lower extremities. *Onchocerca* is also acquired in Africa, and causes river blindness. *Ascaris* is an enteric worm that can cause bowel obstruction or eosinophilic pneumonia.

35. **a) Chancre.** This is the finding in primary syphilis. Congenital syphilis causes the other findings.

36. **e) Cholecystitis.** Group A Strep (*S. pyogenes*) is not a cause of cholecystitis, which is typically caused by enteric anaerobes and gram negative rods. Each of the other diseases are caused by Group A Strep.

37. **b) Molecular mimicry.** Molecular mimicry occurs when the immune system is stimulated by certain cross-reactive foreign antigens. The activated immune system then accidentally recognizes a host antigen of similar structure and starts to attack the host. ADCC occurs when an antibody provides selective targeting of phagocytes toward microbes. Angioedema causes blood vessel and tissue swelling, and is a form of hypersensitivity, or it can be congenital (due to a defect in a complement factor). Anergy occurs when a T cell recognizes its cognate ligand but is turned off, rather than being turned on. Hybridomas are fused human myeloma cells with mouse B cells, allowing immortalization of antibody producing B cells; ultimately this is how monoclonal antibodies are made.

38. **1-d, 2-e, 3-b, 4-c, 5-a.** *Anopheles* mosquitoes carry the agents of malaria. The Reduviid bug transmits Chagas disease (*T. cruzi*). The African tsetse fly carries sleeping sickness (*T. gambiense* or *rhodesiense*). The sandfly transmits *Leishmania*. The *Ixodes* tick transmits Lyme disease (*Borrelia burgdorferi*).

39. **e) 40.** HPV 16, 18, 31, 33, and 35 have been linked to cervical cancer.

40. **b)** *M. marinum.* The patient has fish-tank granuloma. TB, leprosy, and sporotrichosis can all cause skin lesions/granulomas, however the compelling key word is the fish tank exposure. *Nocardia* is an infection that occurs in immunocompromised patients (typically those on steroids), and presents with pneumonia and often brain abscesses.

41. **c) Ammonium magnesium phosphate stone**. The organism is most likely *Proteus*, which produces a urease and splits urea into ammonium, creating a high pH and the appropriate conditions for ammonium magnesium phosphate stone formation. Marble would be very unlikely.

42. **1-d, 2-c, 3-a, 4-b.** IgM has low affinity, but it makes up for it by joining at its Fc region into pentamers, which therefore have 5-fold higher avidity. IgG is the standard immunoglobulin produced during a mature immune response, and is the only subtype that crosses the placenta. IgE is produced during allergic reactions. IgA is transferred across mucosal surfaces to provide protection against adherent microbes.

43. **1-b, 2-c, 3-e, 4-a, 5-d.**

44. **d)** *Legionella.* Any community acquired pneumonia pathogen can cause pneumonia accompanied by high LDH and low sodium. However, for the purposes of the Boards, an extremely high LDH and low sodium in the context of community acquired pneumonia suggests *Legionella*. Furthermore, pneumonia in the context of diarrhea should also suggest *Legionella*, and a pulse-fever dissociation has been described during *Legionella* infection as well. *S. pyogenes* is a very rare cause of pneumonia. *Mycoplasma* on the Boards may present as a "walking pneumonia" in a young adult, often in a military barracks or a college dormitory. *S. aureus* causes pneumonia post-influenza, or from lung seeding during endocarditis or bacteremia, or in patients on a ventilator. TB typically causes upper lobe infiltrates.

45. **d) Agar with iron and cysteine supplementation.** These supplements are necessary to grow *Legionella*. Thayer Martin agar is chocolate agar with antibiotics, and it is used to grow *Neisseria* from a non-sterile site. The antibiotics suppress non-*Neisseria* normal flora. Maconkey agar is used to detect lactose fermenting gram negative rods of the Enterobacteriacea family. Factor V (NAD) and Factor X (heme) are necessary to grow *Hemophilus influenza*. Bordet-Gengou agar is used to grow *Bordetella pertussis*.

46. **b)** *Pseudomonas.* *Pseudomonas* is by far the most common cause of malignant otitis externa in diabetics. The other organisms are common causes of otitis media.

47. **1-e, 2-b, 3-c, 4-a, 5-d.** Reactivation of Varicella Zoster virus causes the dermatomal pain and vesicles seen in Zoster. One of the many syndromes Coxsackie virus can cause is herpangina (pharyngitis with

vesicles). Norwalk virus is a major cause of cruise-ship associated gastroenteritis. Parainfluenza virus causes croup, or tracheobronchitis in children. Human Herpes Virus 8 is associated with Kaposi's sarcoma, largely seen in HIV patients.

48. **b) *Pneumocystis*.** This is the classic presentation of *Pneumocystis* pneumonia in an AIDS patient. CMV rarely causes pneumonitis in HIV; CMV pneumonitis is almost always seen in transplant patients. Lymphoma would not present with diffuse bilateral interstitial infiltrates. Kaposi's sarcoma does cause pulmonary disease, but the chest x-ray findings are atypical, and Kaposi's in the lung is almost always associated with skin and/or mucosal disease. *Aspergillus* may rarely occur in HIV. The bottom line is that if you see 100 patients that present like this, 99 of them will have *Pneumocystis*.

49. **c) *Cryptococcus*.** A high opening pressure in a lumbar puncture from an AIDS patient with low CD4 count is almost always due to *Cryptococcus*. The India ink test is highly specific for *Cryptococcus*. None of the other fungi would be confused with *Cryptococcus* by the India ink test.

50. **d) Trimethoprim-sulfamethoxazole + azithromycin.** Trimethoprim-sulfamethoxazole prophylaxes against both *Pneumocystis* and *Toxoplasma*. Azithromycin prophylaxes against *Mycobacterium avium intracellulare*. There is absolutely no indication to administer levofloxacin or chloroquine to this patient.

INDEX

Note: Page numbers followed by *f* refer to figures; those followed by *t* refer to tables.